Advances in Wound Care, volume I

Other titles available from Wounds UK include:

Honey: A modern wound management product
edited by Richard White, Rose Cooper and Peter Molan

Essential Wound Management: An introduction for undergraduates
edited by David Gray, Pam Cooper and John Timmons

Wound Healing: A systematic approach to advanced wound healing and management edited by David Gray and Pam Cooper

Skin Care in Wound Management: Assessment, prevention and treatment
edited by Richard White

A Pocket Guide to Clinical Decision-making in Wound Management
edited by Sue Bale and David Gray

Paediatric Skin and Wound Care edited by Richard White
and Jacqueline Denyer

Trauma and Pain in Wound Care edited by Richard White
and Keith Harding

Leg Ulcers and Problems of the Lower Limb: An holistic approach edited by
Ellie Lindsay and Richard White

Advances in Wound Care, volume I

edited by
Richard White

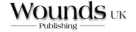
Wounds UK
Publishing

HealthComm UK Limited, trading as Wounds UK Limited, Suite 3.1,
36 Upperkirkgate, Aberdeen AB10 1BA

British Library Cataloguing-in-Publication Data
A catalogue record is available for this book

Printed in the UK by WACE Corporate Print Limited, Swindon, Wiltshire

CONTENTS

Section II: Wound pain and palliative care

Section III: Scientific developments

CONTRIBUTORS

Claire Acton is Tissue Viability and Vascular Nurse Specialist, Surgical Directorate, Queen Elizabeth II Hospital, Greenwich, London

Pauline Beldon is Tissue Viability Nurse Consultant, Epsom and St Helier University Hospitals NHS Trust

Janice Bianchi is Lecturer in Tissue Viability, Glasgow Caledonian University, Glasgow

Natasha Browne is Postgraduate Research Student, Florence Nightingale School of Nursing and Midwifery, King's College, London

Fiona Burton is Tissue Viability Nurse Consultant, University Hospitals Coventry and Warwickshire NHS Trust

Pam Cooper is Clinical Nurse Specialist in Tissue Viability, Grampian Acute Health Services, Aberdeen

Rose Cooper is Reader in Microbiology, University of Wales Institute, Cardiff (UWIC)

Sarah Cowley is Professor in Community Practice Development, Florence Nightingale School of Nursing and Midwifery, King's College, London

Keith Cutting is Principal Lecturer, Buckingham Chilterns University College, High Wycombe and Chalfont St Giles, Buckinghamshire

David Gray is Clinical Nurse Specialist in Tissue Viability, Grampian Acute Health Services, Aberdeen and Clinical Director, Wounds UK, Aberdeen

Patricia Grocott is Senior Fellow, Florence Nightingale School of Nursing and Midwifery, King's College, London

Emma Johnston is Tissue Viability Dietitian, Ulster Community and Hospitals Trust, Northern Ireland

Jane McManus is Deputy Ward Manager, Rugby Ward, St Christopher's Hospice, London

Christine Moffatt is Professor of Nursing and Director of the Centre for Research and Implementation of Clinical Practice (CRICP) at Thames Valley University, London

Olusola Okhiria is a Postgraduate Research Student, University of Wales Institute, Cardiff (UWIC)

Kathy Radley is Clinical Nurse Specialist Dermatology, United Lincolnshire Hospitals NHS Trust

Patricia O'Regan is College Lecturer in the School of Nursing and Midwifery, University College, Cork, Ireland

Andy Roden is Lecturer, Faculty of Health, University of Wales, Bangor

Elaine Shaw is Clinical Nurse Specialist, Tissue Viability, United Lincolnshire Hospitals NHS Trust

Angela Vujnovich is Lead Nurse Stoma Care, St Marks and Northwick Park Hospital, Harrow, Middlesex

Richard White is Professor of Tissue Viability, Institute of Health, Social Care and Psychology, University of Worcester, Worcester

Trudie Young is Lecturer, School of Healthcare Sciences, University of Wales, Bangor

FOREWORD

This book addresses many of the complex issues facing practitioners who are treating patients with all types of wounds and stomas. The diversity of topics covered reflects the many problems that must be faced if successful management is to be employed and considers the developments in practice that have occurred over the last decade.

The first chapter addresses the issue of management of cellulitis in the lower limb. There is increasing evidence that this is costly in terms of use of health service resources and the impact it has on the patient. The second chapter covers the appropriate use of topical steroids for venous ulcer patients. Skin problems are often the most pervasive problem and can delay healing by many months. Appropriate use of topical steroids can bring a rapid resolution to many of these issues, but must be used judiciously with an appreciation of the effect of potency, withdrawal of treatment and the importance of ensuring other concurrent aspects of care such as compression are being used. The chapter on alternatives to the use of Doppler ultrasound in assessment is a welcome addition. While Doppler ultrasound to record an ankle to brachial pressure index (ABPI) remains the gold standard of assessment, there are many instances when the results from this investigation are unreliable, such as the patient with calcified vessels or gross oedema. In these situations other types of investigations such as pulse oximetry can be helpful, and, with a careful clinical history, provide an appropriate level of assessment to allow treatment to commence.

Pressure ulceration remains a growing national and international concern that is set to increase in complexity. The effects of an ageing population and problems such as gross obesity add to this dilemma. *Chapter 4* highlights how best practice in assessment and management of pressure ulceration can significantly alter this situation. Another important aspect of pressure ulcer prevention is covered in the chapter on optimising nutrition in pressure ulcer prevention. Many patients who develop pressure ulceration are malnourished and fail to achieve effective wound healing. Aspects of nutrition and wound healing are often poorly understood and practitioners are frequently ill-equipped to address these issues. The advice given in this chapter will help to redress this issue.

Chronic oedema is now being recognised as a frequent accompaniment to many different wound types and can significantly delay healing. This chapter explains why chronic oedema develops and how this is linked to the different problems associated with wound healing. It is very welcome to see a chapter addressing stoma-related skin problems and management. This topic is often not included in wound text books and yet is a constant challenge to practitioners.

The last two decades have focused on the management of chronic wounds, with complete healing being seen as the only legitimate outcome of treatment. However, for patients with palliative needs, healing is no longer the goal. The chapters in the section on 'Wound pain and palliative care' are invaluable. They will help to focus the practitioner on the control of symptoms such as pain or exudate management that can overwhelm a patient and yet with appropriate management can be controlled. In many situations, symptom control becomes the primary goal of treatment.

The final section of this book covers some of the scientific developments in the field of wound healing. There is much interest in the role of infection and nothing could be more topical in a health service where control of infection is one of the most significant challenges. The chapter on biofilms in wounds will help practitioners understand the complex problems that exist in identifying whether a wound is infected and deciding on treatment strategies. The following chapter on critical colonisation in wounds aids this discussion further. The final chapter of the book is based on inspirational research undertaken by Patricia Grocott that shows how a research-based approach can lead to significant changes in methods of dressing design and production. This work is based on a clear understanding of the clinical and patient problems associated with poor exudate control, particularly in complex situations such as the palliative arena. This chapter also demonstrates how nurses can be at the forefront of wound healing research.

The combined chapters of this book will provide a useful resource to many practitioners working in different healthcare settings with a wide array of patients. Its appeal is the diversity of topics that are covered that reflect the current, real life challenges of everyday practice. I hope you enjoy it.

Professor Christine Moffatt CBE
October 2007

Section I: Aspects of ulceration, oedema and stoma care

CHAPTER 1

MANAGEMENT OF LOWER LIMB CELLULITIS

Pauline Beldon and Fiona Burton

Cellulitis, a deep soft tissue infection, is a common diagnosis made by clinicians. In some patients, however, it may be misdiagnosed since pre-existing chronic diseases such as acute venous insufficiency (Dupuy *et al*, 1999) or acute onset cardiac failure, can result in similar signs and symptoms.

Similarly, erysipelas is a condition which presents as a superficial tissue infection, often affecting only the dermal tissues, causing large areas of painful blistering (*Figure 1.1*). Differential diagnosis can be difficult in both these conditions and can be further complicated by acute problems such as venous thrombosis (Cantrell and Norman, 1998).

Many patients are still unnecessarily admitted to hospital with a diagnosis of cellulitis when, provided prompt action is taken, they could be successfully treated at home. The guidelines presented in this chapter aim to help the practitioner make clear treatment choices, based on a thorough assessment of the patient and differentiation of symptoms.

Erysipelas

Erysipelas is an acute superficial infection, the first symptoms of which are a flu-like general malaise, shivering, and fever. After a few hours the affected area becomes red and epidermal blistering occurs and then spreads with a well-defined advancing edge (Hughes and Van Onselen, 2001; Hunter *et al*, 2002). Erysipelas has been found to occur most frequently among the elderly population (Eriksson *et al*, 1998). Lower limb ulceration has been found to exist in 67% of patients admitted with erysipelas in a study of 229 patients (Erikson *et al*, 1996).

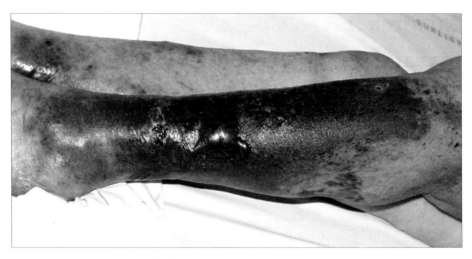

Figure 1.1: Blistering cellulitis

Cellulitis

Cellulitis is defined as a bacterial infection which occurs when bacteria invade the soft tissues through small wounds or abrasions on the skin surface often resulting from an existing condition, eg. leg ulceration or tinea pedis (Hughes and Van Onselen, 2001). Cellulitis extends deeper into the dermis than erysipelas and may involve subcutaneous tissue. The area may be raised as a result of oedema and the erythema is not clearly demarcated, as it is with erysipelas (Hunter *et al*, 2002).

Baddour and Bisno (1982) first described recurrent cellulitis as a previously unreported complication of coronary bypass grafting; they discussed five patients who had 20 episodes of cellulitis occurring in the lower extremity upon which saphenous venectomy had been performed. They suggested that if lymphatic drainage is impaired, this appears to provide a static pool of protein-rich lymph; an excellent medium for bacterial growth.

In a further paper, Baddour and Bisno (1984) noted that although many of the patients observed produced clinical symptoms consistent with infection, eg. pyrexia and rigor, in only three instances ($n = 23$ patients with more than 50 episodes) were α-haemolytic streptococci isolated. They postulated that bacterial toxins which were 'pooled' in poorly drained lymphatic tissue were responsible for these symptoms. This was further explained by Streilan (1984), who stated that the marked inflammatory response of cellulitis was attributable to the dendritic Langerhans cells in the epidermis, which release cytokines, such as interleukin-1 and tumour necrosis factor, when exposed to bacteria. The cytokines clear the bacteria but, in doing so, increase the inflammatory response.

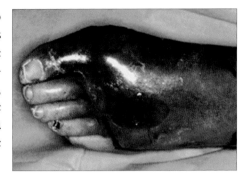

Figure 1.2: Cellulitis preceeded by a traumatic wound on the foot

The causes of cellulitis and erysipelas

Clinical infections are caused by micro-organisms which evade the host's immunological defences on entering a breach in skin integrity and then establish themselves within the tissue of the host where they multiply successfully (Gould, 1994).

Obesity, lymphoedema and pre-existing leg ulceration are all risk factors associated with the conditions. Both cellulitis and erysipelas are often preceded by a history of trauma (*Figure 1.2*), abrasion, skin ulceration (*Figure 1.3*), or an insect bite (El-Daher and Magnussen, 1996) (*Figure 1.4*); although some patients cannot recall any skin injury. Another condition which frequently precedes cellulitis or erysipelas is tinea pedis (Athlete's foot) (Dupuy *et al*, 1999), which, encouraged by moisture, leads to a breach in skin integrity, resulting in toe-web intertrigo.

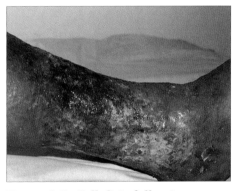

Figure 1.3: Cellulitis following infection of a venous leg ulcer

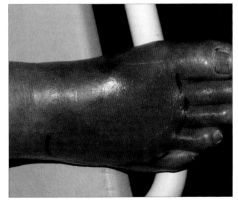

Figure 1.4: Cellulitis following an insect bite to the dorsum of the foot

Common pathogenic causes of cellulitis/erysipelas

The location of the cellulitis on the body will usually be linked to the microbiological cause, eg. cellulitis of the groin is most likely to be caused by anaerobic bacteria (Brook and Frazier, 1995). The bacterial cause of cellulitis may also be haemolytic streptococci, staphylococci, or aerobic or anaerobic gram-negative bacteria.

In those patients with traumatic injury, group A haemolytic streptococci has been identified as the most common pathogen to cause erysipelas, although groups G, C and B and occasionally staphylococci may also be responsible (Bisno and Stevens, 1996).

Conditions which may be mistaken for cellulitis/erysipelas

It is unfortunate that the symptoms of infection which lead to cellulitis and erysipelas are so similar to those of other conditions: erythema, heat, oedema and pain, associated pyrexia, and raised white cell count are often seen. Allergic contact dermatitis (*Figure 1.5*) is caused by sensitisation resulting from exposure to an allergen, while irritant dermatitis is caused by exposure to a substance that damages the normal barrier function of the skin. Both of these conditions may cause inflammation, oedema, pain and exudate leading to misdiagnosis (English, 1997). In both eczema and contact dermatitis, erythema (caused by dilated blood vessels) and blistering (caused by oedema between epidermal cells and within them) result in excessive production of keratin and thickening of the epidermis, both of which are commonly seen in venous insufficiency (Baker *et al*, 1991). Patients with leg ulcers often develop contact dermatitis as a result of the large variety of wound management products, various bandages and the use of latex gloves (Tavadia *et al*, 2003). Every effort should be taken during the treatment of patients with leg ulcers to minimise contact with possible allergens, including latex gloves (Gooptu and Powell, 1999).

Patients with pressure ulcers to the heel who develop persistent

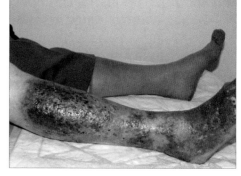

Figure 1.5: Allergic contact dermatitis of right lower leg

cellulitis may have underlying osteomyelitis and should undergo X-ray and possibly bone scan (Sugarman, 1983). More rarely, cellulitis has been reported following pelvic surgery such as vulvectomy (Bouma and Dankert, 1988) or hysterectomy with lymphadenectomy (Dankert and Bouma, 1987), or following pelvic irradiation (Chmel and Hamdy, 1984). However, it is possible that such patients were suffering from acute venous insufficiency, secondary to damage to the lymphatic circulation (Pierce and Daigird, 1991).

Trends in hospital admissions due to cellulitis

Examining the trends of incidence of cellulitis via HES online™ which details hospital episode statistics provides valuable information and provokes questions into the rise of incidence of cellulitis. *Table 1.1* is a collation of pertinent facts regarding cellulitis.

The mean age of those developing cellulitis has changed little in eight years. *Figure 1.6* demonstrates the rise, year on year, in episodes of cellulitis in England. Unfortunately, the statistics do not allow the reader to discriminate between whether these were true cases of infective cellulitis or that caused by obesity, lymphoedema or lower limb dependency. *Figure 1.7* shows there is no obvious tendency towards the development of cellulitis in either gender.

Table 1.1: Statistics relating to cellulitis hospital admissions							
Year	Number of admissions to hospital	Number of episodes	Male	Female	Mean length of stay	Mean age	Number of bed days
1998/9	33903	40792	20138	20654	8.5	57	280546
1999/0	37833	46041	22871	23170	8.5	57	312111
2000/1	41100	51411	25429	25982	8.7	57	351765
2001/2	42308	54040	26654	27386	8.9	57	367510
2002/3	45123	59004	29537	29467	9.3	58	403700
2003/4	49491	66268	33550	32718	9	60	425804
2004/5	51551	69576	35497	34079	8.3	60	429811
2005/6	53952	74247	37592	36655	8	60	425610

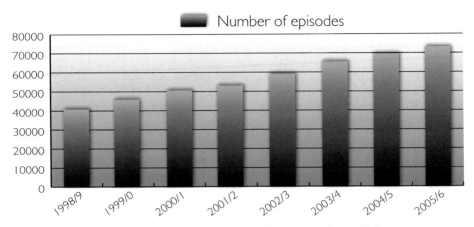

Figure 1.6: Number of recorded hospital admissions for cellulitis

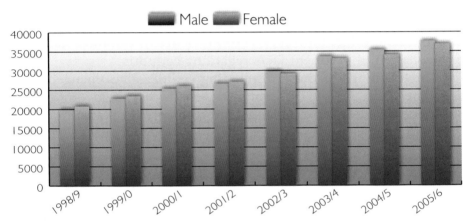

Figure 1.7: Numbers of male/female patients admitted to hospital with dangerous cellulitis

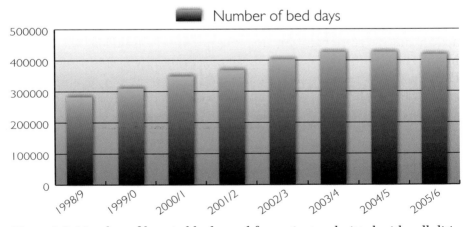

Figure 1.8: Number of hospital beds used for patients admitted with cellulitis

The average length of stay in hospital is currently eight days (Hospital Episodes Statistics [HES], 2007; *Figure 1.8*), this equates to the number of bed days used by patients with a diagnosis of cellulitis being in excess of 400 000 per year. Since the main aims of treatment are pain relief, antibiotic therapy, elevation of limb and skin care, practitioners should be asking themselves whether these bed days are necessary, or would it not be better for the patient and the health service if a large proportion of these patients were cared for in primary care settings. It should only be those patients that are acutely unwell who are admitted to secondary care.

Lower limb cellulitis algorithms

Patients with a diagnosis of cellulitis are encountered on a regular basis in both primary and secondary care. It is important that nurses working in primary care recognise the symptoms of cellulitis and so a correct diagnosis can be made and appropriate management commenced early. This will help to minimise pain and distress for the patient and prevent the need for admission to secondary care. It will also avoid the patient's condition being misdiagnosed and so prevent the unnecessary use of antibiotics.

The lower limb cellulitis algorithms (*Figures 1.9* and *1.10*) are recommended as an aid to differential diagnosis to help ensure that patients receive the appropriate medical and nursing care that they deserve. The algorithm should be used in conjunction with a thorough nursing assessment of the patient.

Immediate nursing management of cellulitis is dependent upon first recognising the cause of the problem by conducting an accurate patient assessment. Once a diagnosis of cellulitis has been made, nursing action may vary depending on whether the cellulitis is wet or dry, however, in both instances the patient will require systemic antibiotic therapy. The common treatment for both wet or dry cellulitis is a combination of benzylpenicillin (unless contraindicated by allergy), and a broad-spectrum antibiotic such as flucloxicillin, which is active against both streptococci and staphylococci. Antibiotics may be given intravenously initially and then orally once a therapeutic effect is noted, ie. a reduction in white cell count (Baxter and McGregor, 2001). Wound swabs should be obtained from the affected area or limb if there is exudate present in order to determine both the causative organism and sensitivity to antibiotic therapy (Holzapel *et al*, 1999).

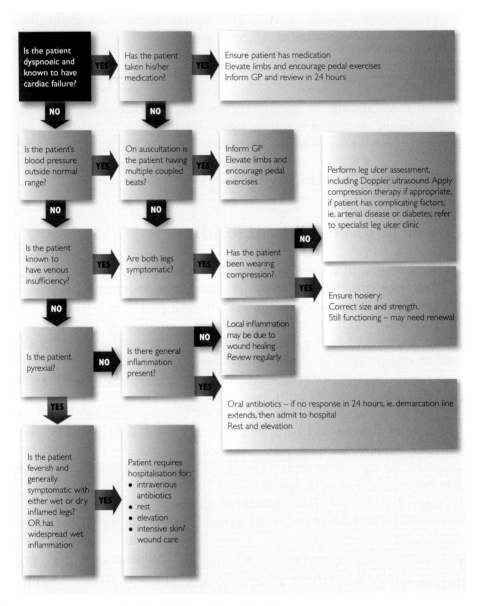

Figure 1.9: Lower limb cellulitis algorithm for primary care

Managing dry cellulitis

A wound with dry cellulitis (*Figure 1.11*) should remain so and not be cleansed. The affected area or limb will react as an erythematous burn injury and will be oedematous, acutely painful and inflamed.

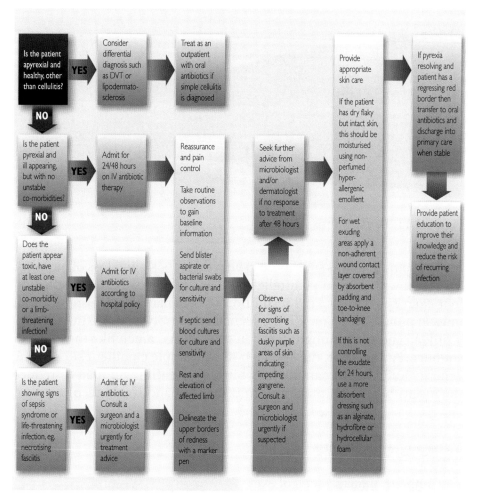

Figure 1.10: Lower limb cellulitis algorithm for secondary care

The demarcated area of cellulitis should be outlined with a skin marker pen (*Figure 1.12*), as an indicator of whether the cellulitis is resolving or extending. The patient's symptoms should guide treatment. Pain management is the priority as any affected patient will say. Analgesia must always be taken regularly and patients may need this reinforcing; elderly patients especially are not enthusiastic about analgesia (Gloth, 2000).

Elevation is key to reducing oedema, and patients should be encouraged to rest with the affected area raised. Bed rest, with the foot of the bed elevated, may be necessary, although elderly patients especially should still be encouraged to mobilise in order to avoid

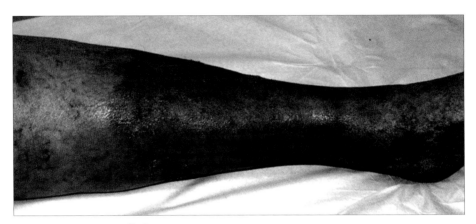

Figure 1.11: Dry cellulitis

further complications such as deep vein thrombosis and loss of mobility. Elevation will also aid pain relief as the oedema resolves. Dorsiflexion foot exercises will also aid resolution of oedema by activating the calf muscle pump (Hofman, 1998). As oedema resolves, the skin becomes wrinkled and often sloughs away in thin sheets, much like the effect of sunburn. At this time, the application of a simple emollient such as the generic 50/50 liquid paraffin in white soft paraffin will help to reduce the insensible loss of moisture from the skin and so aid recovery.

Managing wet cellulitis

The nursing management of wet cellulitis is more problematic. As with dry cellulitis, analgesia is vital to enable the patient to participate in his/her care and the affected area or limb also requires elevation. Control of exudate to reduce the effects of maceration is often difficult and may require the use of absorbent dressings, ie. foams, hydrofibres, or alginates. These will require very frequent changes in the initial period of treatment since there is a danger that once the primary dressing

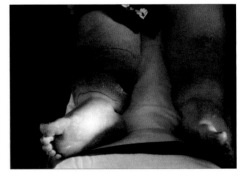

Figure 1.12: A skin marker pen has been used to identify the border of cellulitis to enable clinicians to determine whether treatment is successful in resolving infection

is saturated with exudate, the surrounding skin will become affected. An alternative is to use a non-adherent contact layer, ie. Mepitel™ (Mölnlycke Health Care, UK), N/A Ultra™ (Johnson and Johnson, UK), or Urgotulle™ (Laboratoires Urgo, France) and to leave this in situ while changing the outer dressing. This may be more comfortable for the patient and prove cost-effective.

The effectiveness of potassium permanganate soaks as an astringent and weak antiseptic is debatable and there are no randomised controlled trials examining its effectiveness. If using potassium permanganate, care must be taken to obtain the correct dilution of 1:10,000. Instruction is generally given to dilute until a 'rose-pink' colour is obtained. In addition, there have been instances of skin irritation caused by potassium permanganate solution (Hughes and Van Onselen, 2001), although this may have been caused by use of a stronger than directed dilution.

Long-term treatment of cellulitis

Once the initial period of infection has subsided, the skin of the affected area may still require treatment with an emollient for several weeks in order to regain normal elasticity and integrity. Scarring and permanent 'tattooing' of the skin is not uncommon, although in most instances this will fade in time. Care should be taken to avoid exposure to the sun or trauma as the new skin will remain delicate for several weeks (Baxter and McGregor, 2001).

In addition, the patient may need to wear compression hosiery to prevent a recurrence if the initial trigger has been venous disease and ulceration. It is also vital that the patient recognises the importance of preventing a recurrence and understands how he/she can take responsibility for this prevention. Patient information sheets are valuable to reinforce information and to act as a prompt.

Conclusion

Cellulitis must be identified by a knowledgeable practitioner who is able to instigate the correct treatment and to identify when the underlying cause is not infection, but a concurrent disease. Use of guidelines helps to standardise practice and disseminate knowledge of a disorder, giving both the practitioner and the patient confidence in both the outcome of treatment and the prevention of recurrence.

References

Baddour LM, Bisno AL (1984) Recurrent cellulitis after coronary bypass surgery; association with superficial fungal infection in saphenous venectomy limbs. *JAMA* **251**(8): 1049–52

Baker SR, Stacey MC, Joop-McKay AG, Hospkin SE, Thompson PJ (1991) Epidemiology of chronic venous ulcers. *Br J Surg* **78**: 864–7

Baxter H, McGregor F (2001) Understanding and managing cellulitis. *Nurs Standard* **15**(44): 50–6

Bisno AL, Stevens DL (1996) Current concepts: streptococcal infections of the skin and soft tissues. *N Engl J Med* **334**: 240–5

Bouma J, Dankert J (1988) Recurrent acute leg cellulitis in patients after radical vulvectomy. *Gynaecol Oncol* **29**(1): 50–7

Brook I, Frazier EH (1995) Clinical features and aerobic and anaerobic microbiological characteristics of cellulitis. *Arch Surg* **130**(7): 786–92

Cantrell M, Norman DC (1998) Skin and soft tissue infections in the elderly. *Baillière's Clinical Infectious Diseases* **5**(1): 71–81

Chmel H, Hamdy M (1984) Recurrent streptococcal cellulitis complicating radical hysterectomy and radiation therapy. *Obstet Gynaecol* **63**(6): 862–4

Dankert J, Bouma J (1987) Recurrent acute leg cellulitis after hysterectomy with pelvic lymphadenectomy. *Br J Obstet Gynaecol* **94**: 788–90

Dupuy A, Benchikhi H, Roujeau J, *et al* (1999) Risk factors for erysipelas of the leg (cellulitis): case control study. *Br Med J* **318**: 1591–4

El-Daher N, Magnussen CR (1996) Skin and Soft Tissue Infections: Outpatient Management and Indications for Hospitalisation. *Consultant* **36**(12): 2563–6

English JSC (1997) Contact dermatitis. *Medicine* **25**: 42–5

Eriksson B, Jorup-Romstrom C, Karkkonen K, Sjoblom AC, Holm SE (1996) Erysipelas: clinical and bacteriologic spectrum and serological aspects. *Clin Infect Dis* **23**(5): 1091–8

Gloth FM (2000) Geriatric pain: factors that limit pain relief and increase complications. *Geriatrics* **55**(10): 45–50

Gooptu C, Powell SM (1999) The problems of rubber sensitivity (types 1 & IV) in chronic leg ulcer and stasis eczema patients. *Contact Dermatitis* **41**: 89–93

Gould D (1994) Infection control. Understanding the nature of bacteria. *Nurs Standard* **8**(28): 29–31

Greenberg J, DeSanctis RW, Mills RM (1982) Vein donor leg cellulitis after coronary artery bypass surgery. *Ann Intern Med* **97**: 565–6

HES online™ Hospital Episodes Statistics. Available online at: <u>www. hesonline.nhs.uk/Ease/servlet/ContentServer?siteID=1937&categoryID= 203</u> (last accessed 2 September 2007)

Hughes E, Van Onselen J, eds (2001) *Dermatology Nursing; a Practical Guide*. Churchill Livingstone, London: 207

Hofman D (1998) Oedema and the management of venous leg ulcers. *J Wound Care* 7(7): 345–8

Holzapel L, Jacquet-Francillon T, Rahmani J, *et al* (1999) Microbiological evaluation of infected wounds of the extremities in 214 adults. *J Acc Emerg Med* **16**: 32–4

Hunter J, Savin J, Dahl M (2002) *Clinical Dermatology*. 3rd edn. Blackwell Science Ltd, Oxford, London: 192–3

Pierce RP, Daigird AJ (1991) Recurrent leg cellulitis: pathogenesis, treatment and prevention. *J Am Board Family Pract* **5**(1): 85–7

Sugarman B, Hawes S, Mushner D (1983) Osteomyelitis beneath pressure sores. *Arch Intern Med* **143**(4): 683

Tavadia S, Bianchi J, Dawe RS, *et al* (2003) Allergic contact dermatitis in venous leg ulcer patients. *Contact Dermatitis* **48**(5): 261–5

Chapter 2

Topical corticosteroids and their use in venous leg ulcers

Kathy Radley and Elaine Shaw

This chapter addresses the use of topical corticosteroids in venous leg ulcers to make readers aware of the two most likely reasons for eczema associated with venous leg ulcers and enable their identification and appropriate treatment. Although significant advances have been made in the management of lower limb ulceration and in the understanding of its causative factors, venous ulceration of the lower leg continues to place an enormous burden on patients and healthcare resources (Moffatt *et al*, 1992).

In the UK, it is estimated that the cost to the NHS of managing venous leg ulcers is between £236–600m per year (Freak *et al*, 1996). With a prevalence rate that exceeds 15% in the over-65s (Grundy, 1992), and an ever-increasing elderly population, it is unlikely that this cost will be substantially reduced.

Approximately 70% of all venous ulceration is caused by venous insufficiency associated with chronic venous hypertension. A further 10% are arterial and are caused by peripheral arterial disease, thrombosis or compromised microcirculation due to rheumatoid arthritis, diabetes or autoimmune diseases. A combination of arterial and venous incompetence accounts for 15% of cases and a further 5% are a result of more unusual causes (Nelzen *et al*, 1991). Even with major advancements in treatment, leg ulcers remain difficult to heal, painful, debilitating and have a significant impact on quality of life.

The two main reasons for the use of topical corticosteroids in venous ulcers are gravitational eczema (also called venous, varicose or stasis eczema) and allergic contact dermatitis (ACD). However, a patient's lower limb should never be treated in isolation and there may be other dermatoses to be considered such as atopic eczema, psoriasis or cellulitis. With both gravitational eczema and ACD, simply treating the presenting eczema alone will not alleviate the underlying cause.

Crucially, healthcare professionals need to involve patients in their care to improve treatment compliance (Nursing and Midwifery Council [NMC], 2004). Patients need to understand their condition and its likely causes and treatments. One of the symptoms of untreated eczema, regardless of the cause, is itching. It is important to explain how scratching can exacerbate the eczema and cause further damage. Using distraction techniques when itching occurs, or minimising damage, eg. by rubbing with a finger rather than scratching with nails, can help.

Gravitational eczema

Gravitational eczema occurs due to venous insufficiency and venous hypertension (*Figure 2.1*). The exact inflammatory mechanism within the skin is not known, but inflammation is produced by the skin's immune cells activated by cytokine release. Accumulation of the inflammatory cells leads to the clinical changes present in eczematous skin. As discussed later in the chapter, oedema due to increased capillary pressure and the presence of proteolytic enzymes also contribute to these changes. Gravitational eczema is an endogenous eczema.

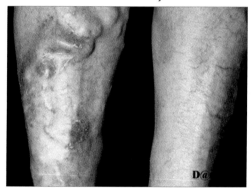

Figure 2.1: A patient with gravitational eczema

To understand why venous ulceration and gravitational eczema occur, a basic understanding of the mechanics of venous return and the anatomy of venous circulation is essential. Return of venous blood from the lower limb is a complex mechanism, which relies on the deep, superficial and perforator veins to work in combination with the calf muscle pump, ie:

- *Deep veins:* these consist of both popliteal and femoral veins surrounded by muscle. They lie deep within the fascia, carry blood at high pressure and contain few valves.
- *Superficial veins:* these consist of both long and short saphenous veins that lie outside the fascia. They are unsupported by muscle,

carry blood under low pressure and contain a series of valves to prevent backflow.

- *Perforator veins:* these link the deep and superficial systems and pass through the deep fascia. They are relatively thick-walled vessels, which also contain a series of valves to prevent backflow from the deep system to the superficial.

Venous ulcers are caused by a failure of one or all of these mechanisms to return the blood back to the heart efficiently. The interconnecting layout of these veins is shown in *Figure 2.2* (Orr and McAvoy, 1987).

As the venous system has no autonomic pump, the veins must rely primarily on the action of the calf muscle. Through dorsiflexion, the calf muscle compresses a segment of deep vein, forcing the blood upwards and out of the vein with backflow prevented by the valves. The empty segment of vein refills with blood from the superficial system and the cycle is repeated.

Aetiology of venous hypertension and ulceration

In normal veins, the flow of blood is upwards towards the heart with the presence of valves preventing backflow. In venous hypertension, abnormally high pressures are transmitted to the superficial and capillary system when valve failure in the perforator vessels allows reverse blood flow.

Normal capillary pressure is in the region of 25–30 mmHg. When damage in the vein has occurred, blood flows in the wrong direction through the vein. As this progresses over time, the pressure can rise to over 90mmHg.

The capillaries, in an attempt to compensate for this increase in pressure, become tortuous and

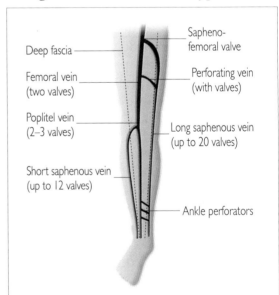

Figure 2.2: The layout of veins in the lower leg

Deep fascia

Sapheno-femoral valve

Femoral vein (two valves)

Perforating vein (with valves)

Poplitel vein (2–3 valves)

Long saphenous vein (up to 20 valves)

Short saphenous vein (up to 12 valves)

Ankle perforators

dilated, allowing abnormal amounts of fluid to leak into the interstitial space, resulting in oedema. The presence of proteolytic enzymes in this fluid act as an irritant and contribute to the presence of gravitational eczema, which is often associated with venous hypertension and the resulting venous leg ulcers. Also, red cells leak out from these dilated vessels, depositing their haem content into the interstitial spaces, resulting in brown staining of the skin (haemosiderin staining).

In conjunction with venous hypertension, there are thought to be other processes that contribute to the development of ulceration, such as fibrin cuff theory and white cell trapping. Fibrin cuff theory occurs when leakage of plasma into the soft tissues deposits fibrin that surrounds the capillaries. This fibrin resembles a rubber band and forms a constricting cuff around the capillary, creating a diffusion barrier. Oxygen and nutrients are prevented from reaching the skin and waste products and water cannot be removed.

As a result of this, the skin and veins supplying the skin become affected, manifesting in the patient's leg feeling hard, fibrous and indurated. This process is known as lipodermatosclerosis (Burnand *et al*, 1982).

White cell trapping occurs when the patient's capillaries become blocked by white cells that are trapped between the capillary walls, leading to limited oxygen delivery to the tissues, contributing to skin breakdown (Coleridge Smith *et al*, 1988).

The debate, however, continues regarding the extent of the effect these two processes have on the development of ulceration. Studies would suggest that these two theories are, in fact, actually describing different aspects in a sequence of events (Herrick *et al*, 1992).

Assessment

For effective management to take place, a true aetiology of the ulcer must be first established by undertaking a full holistic assessment to identify risk factors such as age, gender, cardiovascular disease, body mass index (BMI), mobility, arthritis, diabetes and any previous history of deep vein thrombosis (DVT), varicose vein surgery or leg injury.

Ulcers of a venous or mixed aetiology usually present in conjunction with signs of venous hypertension, such as lipodermatosclerosis, pigmentation, superficial varicosities, oedema, eczema, atrophy blanche and ankle flare. They are usually shallow and irregular in appearance, well vascularised, highly exudating and often very painful.

The site of the ulcer is also another good indicator to the underlying pathology, with a majority of venous ulcers occurring in the gaiter area (Gibson, 1995). If ulceration is present on the foot or the calf, nurses should treat with caution as this may indicate the presence of vasculitis, ischaemia or undiagnosed diabetes.

Along with patient history, Doppler ultrasound is a crucial part of the assessment to detect the presence of arterial impairment. However, it should not be taken in isolation and the Doppler or ankle brachial pressure index (ABPI) reading in conjunction with signal quality and type should merely confirm what the nurse already suspects from the patient history and clinical appearance. The presence of arterial disease (ABPI of <0.8) has an impact on further management strategy and misdiagnosis may have disastrous consequences for patients who have diabetes or a significant arterial deficit. When assessing patients with poorly controlled or advanced diabetes, it should be taken into account that their ABPI may be elevated due to arterial calcification. The result may therefore be unreliable. If in doubt, an onward referral for a surgical opinion should be sought for further investigations.

Management

The effective management of patients with venous leg ulceration and associated gravitational eczema lies in controlling and compensating for the damaged venous system. Sustained graduated compression is a vital component of successful treatment. The precise optimum pressure needed to overcome venous hypertension is not known, but is estimated to be approximately 30–40 mmHg (Stemmer, 1969). Graduated compression systems aim to apply 40 mmHg at the ankle, graduating to 17 mmHg below the knee.

Patients with a mixed aetiology ulcer may be suitable for reduced compression. However, if compression therapy is to be applied, the importance of accurate assessment and diagnosis cannot be overstated.

Sub-bandaging pressures

Graduated compression is achieved by the direct application of external pressure aided by the natural radius of the curvature of the leg. The majority of legs are narrower at the ankle than at the knee, therefore, graduated compression can be achieved naturally if the tension of the bandages are maintained for the length of the leg. The pressure produced by a bandage can be calculated by using Laplace's law, which states (P = sub-bandage pressure; T = tension; N = number of layers; C = limb circumference; W = width of the bandage):

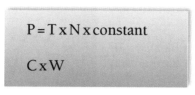

$$P = \frac{T \times N \times constant}{C \times W}$$

These pressures are inversely proportional to the radius of the curvature of the limb. Therefore, to achieve an adequate level of compression, a large limb which is particularly swollen with oedema would require a higher level of compression than a smaller, thinner limb.

Compression therapy is now available in a wide variety of systems; multilayer, long-stretch, short-stretch and two-layer compression hosiery. All of these systems provide therapeutic sub-bandaging pressures. Ultimately, the healthcare professional must assess which system best suits the needs of the individual patient.

Allergic contact dermatitis

ACD is an exogenous eczema and is an acquired sensitivity from an external agent (*Figure 2.3*). Some patients may experience an acute reaction after a brief contact with a strong irritant, or with prolonged exposure to weaker irritants. The most common irritants include detergents and alkalis and, while the hands are the most common site, wound exudate can have a similar effect. The correct dressing selection can help to manage this (Hunter *et al*, 1995). Such irritation is not true ACD but would be classed as irritant contact dermatitis.

ACD produces a delayed hypersensitivity. This type-IV reaction is a result of a cell-mediated immune response activated by lymphocytes. Diagnosis of ACD is made by patch testing, although the distribution of the eczema may provide an indicator. Cameron (1998) cites the most common allergens as topical antibiotics and states that the routine use of preparations known as common sensitisers has decreased in recent years. Other common allergens include emulsifiers, stabilisers and rubbers (Patel *et al*, 2001).

A diagnosis of ACD should be suspected if appropriate treatment for a venous ulcer does not result in an improvement in the eczema (especially use of compression if indicated). Nurses need to be aware that this is also true with the use of topical corticosteroids, indeed, the topical treatment may well be the cause of the ACD. Vesicles will also be present. The distribution of the eczema may also indicate ACD, for example, if the cause is a rubber allergy, other sites in contact with rubber will also be affected.

ACD is treated by avoidance of the identified allergen and it is important that patients both understand the cause and how to avoid the allergen. This must

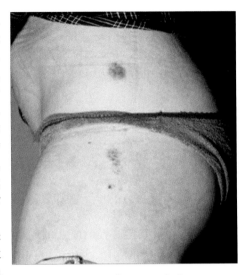

Figure 2.3: ACD from nickel jean studs

also be communicated to all those involved in the patient's care. It is not uncommon for gravitational eczema and ACD to present simultaneously (Patel *et al*, 2001), and the underlying causes for both need to be treated for sustained relief.

Topical corticosteroids

Indications for the use of topical corticosteroids include inflammatory skin disorders, which in turn include both gravitational eczema and ACD (British Medical Association and Royal Pharmaceutical Society of Great Britain [BMA/RPSGB], 2006). Contraindications include untreated bacterial, fungal or viral skin infections, or an ACD reaction to one of the ingredients of the topical corticosteroid. Topical corticosteroids are absorbed through the horny layer of the skin. *Table 2.1* shows their anti-inflammatory and immunosuppressive actions. Preparations of topical corticosteroids are available as creams, ointments and lotions. On dry lesions ointments are the preparation of choice, as absorption is improved due to ease of transfer through the horny layer of the skin.

Creams are more appropriate on wet or weeping lesions. Lotions are usually formulated for use on the scalp, although it should be remembered that while their use is unlikely on venous leg ulcers, they may be appropriate on wounds such as stomas where adhesive dressings are required.

Preparations of topical corticosteroids are classed using four groups of potency (BMA/RPSGB, 2006):

- mild
- potent
- moderate
- very potent

While it is important to use the least potent at the lowest strength whenever possible, the treatment does need to be effective and using a more potent preparation initially may result in less topical corticosteroid being used in the long-term.

Side-effects from the use of topical corticosteroids can be both topical and systemic and are related to potency, with the most potent causing the most side-effects. Systemic side-effects of topical corticosteroids are not common, but a significant absorption of potent or very potent preparations can cause pituitary and adrenal suppression, and Cushing's syndrome.

The most common local side-effect is thinning of the skin. Although the skin may recover thickness after the topical corticosteroid is discontinued, the original structure may never return (National Institute for Health and Clinical Excellence [NICE], 2004). Irreversible loss of elasticity and striae may also occur. Worsening of skin infections or acne can also be present, and, ironically, ACD can be caused by sensitivity to an ingredient in the topical corticosteroid preparation.

Table 2.1: The pharmacological action of topical corticosteroids (Hunter et al, 1995)

Anti-inflammatory:
1. Vasoconstricting
2. Decrease the permeability of dermal vessels
3. Decrease phagocytic migration and activity
4. Decrease fibrin formation
5. Decrease kinin formation
6. Inhibit phospholipase A2 activity and decrease the products of arachidonic acid metabolism
7. Depress fibroblastic activity
8. Stabilise lysosomal membranes

Immunosuppressive:
1. Antigen-antibody interaction is unaffected but inflammatory consequences lessened by above mechanisms and by inhibiting cytokines
2. Lympholytic

Healthcare professionals should be suspicious if the eczema is not responding to treatment.

Side-effects will be more likely on thinner skin, for example, the face, and less likely where the skin is thicker, for example, the palms or soles. This is because thicker layers of skin allow less corticosteroid to be absorbed. Occlusion enhances the potency of topical corticosteroids by aiding absorption and this, together with the frequency of the application, should be considered when choosing an appropriate preparation.

Guidance states that in atopic eczema topical corticosteroids should be applied once or twice-daily (NICE, 2004). However, in the case of gravitational eczema or ACD surrounding a leg ulcer, the ulcer will usually be undergoing treatment by compression therapy and dressing changes will not allow this frequency of application. The frequency of application should also be considered alongside potency.

A useful guide to the amount of topical corticosteroid to be applied is the fingertip unit (FTU) (Long and Finlay, 1991). *Table 2.2* shows the maximum recommended amount of topical corticosteroid per application and is a useful guide to assist in applying the correct amount. It is easier to estimate five FTUs, rather than try and measure 2.5 g from a 50 g tube. As mentioned above, the frequency of dressing changes will also have a considerable effect on the amount of topical corticosteroid used over time.

Table 2.2: The fingertip guide to applying topical corticosteroids	
Fingertip guide – 1 fingertip unit (FTU) = 0.5g	
Average adult (maximum per application)	
Face and neck	= 2 FTU
Trunk, front	= 7 FTU
Trunk, back	= 7 FTU
One arm	= 3 FTU
One hand	= 1 FTU
One leg	= 5 FTU
One foot	= 2 FTU

Other topical treatments

Drying of the skin is part of the normal ageing of the skin and as the demographic data in the introduction shows, ulceration is more prevalent in the older population. The use of topical emollients will help to maintain the skin's function as a barrier as well as providing more comfort for the patient. Greasy emollients can build up under bandages and this does need to be washed off, otherwise emollient and skin cells can form thick greasy flakes. Soap substitutes should be used if necessary to avoid drying the skin further.

Eczema that persists and is particularly itchy can be relieved by using paste bandages. However, these are time-consuming and messy to use and caution must be taken to prevent topical sensitisation causing ACD. Wet, weepy eczema may respond to potassium permanganate solution (0.01%). The affected area should be immersed, or alternatively, gauze can be soaked in the solution and applied (BMA/RPSGB, 2006). It is important to inform patients before use that soaking will stain the toenails — applying nail varnish before beginning the treatment can minimise this. However, some guidelines do note a lack of evidence on the clinical effectiveness of this technique in wounds (Royal College of Nursing [RCN], 2001).

Dressing selection

Accurate wound assessment is crucial and should consider factors such as exudate levels, odour, pain and general wound and peri-wound appearance. To date, no reliable studies have confirmed that more complex dressings offer any advantage over a simple non-adherent dressing type, especially in an uncomplicated venous ulcer in conjunction with graduated compression therapy (Eich and Stadler, 1999).

Conclusion

This chapter has highlighted the most likely causes of eczema surrounding venous leg ulcers and discussed the relevant treatments. However, it is vital not only that the eczema is treated appropriately, but also that the underlying cause is identified and treated accordingly.

All pictures are reproduced with permission from *An Atlas of Clinical Dermatology* by Neils K Veien and Mads Nielsen (D@nderm).

References

British Medical Association and Royal Pharmaceutical Society of Great Britain (2006) *British National Formulary*. BMJ Publishing Group LTD, London

Burnand KG, Whimster I, Naidoo A, Browse NL (1982) Pericapillary fibrin in the ulcer-bearing skin of the leg: the cause of lipodermatosclerosis and venous ulceration. *Br Med J* **285**: 1071–2

Cameron J (1998) Contact sensitivity in patients with leg ulcers. British *J Dermatol Nurs* **2**(4): 5–7

Coleridge Smith PD, Thomas P, Scurr JH, Normandy JA (1988) Causes of venous ulceration: a new hypothesis. *Br Med J* **296**: 1726–7

Eich D, Stadler R (1999) Differentiated local therapy of chronic wounds with modern wound dressings. *Vasa* **28**(1): 3–9

Freak L, Simon D, Kinsella A (1996) Leg ulcer care in the UK: an audit of cost-effectiveness. *Health Trends* **27**: 133–6

Gibson B (1995) The nursing assessment of patients with leg ulcers. In: Cullum N, Roe B, eds. *Leg Ulcers: Nursing Management – A Research-based Guide*. Scutari Press, Harrow

Grundy E (1992) The epidemiology of aging. In: Brockhurst JC, Tallis JC, Fillit HM, eds. *Textbook of Geriatric medicine and Gerontology*. 4th edn. Churchill Livingstone, Edinburgh: 3–20

Herrick SE, Sloan P, McGurk M, Freak L, McCollum CN, Ferguson MWJ (1992) Sequential changes in histological pattern and extracellular matrix deposition during the healing of chronic venous ulcers. *Am J Pathol* **141**: 1085–95

Hunter JAA, Savin JA, Dahl MV (1995) *Clinical Dermatology*. Blackwell Scientific, Oxford

Long CC, Finlay AY (1991) The fingertip unit — a new practical measure. *Clin Exp Dermatol* **16**: 444–7

Moffatt CJ, Franks PJ, Oldroyd MI, *et al* (1992) Community clinics for leg ulcers and impact on healing. *Br Med J* **305**: 1389–92

Nelzen O, Berquist D, Lindhagen A (1991) Leg ulcer aetiology: a cross sectional population study. *J Vasc Surg* **14**(4): 557–64

National Institute for Clinical Excellence (2004) *Technology Appraisal Guidance 81. Frequency of Application of Topical Corticosteroids for Atopic Eczema*. NICE, London

Nursing and Midwifery Council (2004) *Code of Professional Conduct: Standards for Conduct, Performance and Ethics*. NMC, London

Orr MM, McAvoy BR (1987) The ischaemic leg. In: Fry J, Berry HE, eds. *Surgical Problems in Clinical Practice*. Edward Arnold, London: 123–35

Patel GK, Llewellyn M, Harding KG (2001) Managing gravitational eczema and allergic contact dermatitis. *Br J Comm Nurs* **6**(8): 394–406

Royal College of Nursing (2001) *The Management of Patients with Venous Leg Ulcers*. RCN, London

Stemmer R (1969) Ambulatory-elasto-compressive treatment of the lower extremities particularly with elastic stockings. *Derm Kassenarzt* **9**: 1–8

CHAPTER 3

LOI: AN ALTERNATIVE TO DOPPLER IN LEG ULCER PATIENTS

Janice Bianchi

Systematic reviews suggest that compression systems improve the healing of venous leg ulcers and should be used routinely in uncomplicated venous ulcers (Fletcher *et al*, 1997; Cullum *et al*, 2002). Compression treatment of the leg can, however, be hazardous in limbs with occult arterial disease (Callam *et al*, 1987a). In order to exclude significant peripheral arterial disease before applying compression, Doppler ankle brachial pressure index (ABPI) has become the accepted test recommended in recent years (Callam *et al*, 1987a, b; Clinical Resource Efficiency Support Team [CREST], 1998; Royal College of Nursing [RCN], 1998; Scottish Intercollegiate Guidelines Network [SIGN], 1998).

However, the technique requires considerable skill, particularly when locating foot arteries and maintaining the correct probe angle (Ray *et al*, 1994). Strandess *et al* (1967) suggested that in order to ensure reproducibility of the signal when measuring Doppler ABPI, it is important to maintain a constant angle between the probe and the vessel being examined. Others have noted variability between right and left legs, suggesting observers may experience more difficulty measuring one leg than the other, due to the position of the patient and the position of the observer's hand (Fowkes *et al*, 1988; Kaiser *et al*, 1999). Even vascular technicians with specialised skills in Doppler ABPI have had difficulty with the technique, particularly in individuals whose arterial flow was difficult to detect (Fowkes *et al*, 1988). Additionally, Bianchi *et al* (2002) noted that in patients with oedema or lymphoedema the signal can be difficult to detect.

The appropriate period of training in Doppler ABPI has not been determined, however, Ray *et al* (1994) found that an intensive training programme over a six-week period produced less errors in Doppler ABPI examination than a single educational session. However, this extended period of training may only be available to a few practitioners. Maintaining Doppler ABPI skills may also prove difficult for nurses who carry out the test on an irregular basis. Kaiser *et al* (1999) identified experienced recorders of ABPI as those who carry out the procedure more than 10 times a week and the less experienced as those who perform Doppler assessment 5 to 15 times a month. Vowden and Vowden (2002) suggested that anxiety over Doppler assessment is, perhaps, an indication that a change in service management is needed.

The history of pulse oximetry

In reports from as early as 1874, oxygen consumption and arterial occlusion were measured by spectroscopy. According to Severinghaus *et al* (1998), von Vierordt measured oxygen consumption using transmitted light in a crude experiment. Wrapping a rubber band around his wrist to cut off the circulation and shining a light on his hand, he saw that two bands of oxyhaemoglobin disappeared and a band of deoxyhaemoglobin appeared. Using reflected light from a spectrometer, he measured the oxygen consumption of the living tissue by noting the time that elapsed as oxyhaemoglobin changed to deoxyhaemoglobin.

Fifty-five years later and with better equipment, Nicolia resurrected von Vierordt's work. Nicolia added photo-electric light detection and his student, Kramer, introduced the new German barrier-layer photocells to record saturation *in vivo* by transilluminating the arteries of animals (Ridlen, 1998).

In 1935, Mathers built the first device that continuously measured human blood oxygen saturation. He used two wavelengths of light, one that was sensitive to changes of oxygenation and another that was not. This device could follow trends in saturation but was difficult to calibrate (Tremper and Barker, 1989). Squire developed a similar device that was calibrated by compressing the tissue to eliminate the blood (Squire, 1940).

In the early 1940s, Millikan coined the term 'oximeter' to describe a lightweight device he developed for aviation research (Millikan, 1942). Later, when Wood and others used oximeters similar to Millikan's in the operating room, they were noted to detect significant desaturation even during routine anaesthetics (Wood and Geraci,

1949; Stephen *et al*, 1951). Surprisingly, despite being developed over half a century ago, pulse oximeters were only commercially marketed from 1981 onwards (Woodrow, 1999). Initially, the pulse oximeter was confined to use in anaesthetics, intensive care and other emergency situations (Ridlen, 1998), but, by 1986, they were recommended as a standard of care for every patient undergoing general anaesthesia in the USA (Eichorn, 1986).

More recently, their ability to detect tissue perfusion and arterial occlusion pressure has been exploited and has seen them being increasingly used in new and novel ways, from the detection of peripheral neuropathy (Modi *et al*, 1997) to the viability of tissue after surgery (Lindsay *et al*, 1991; Yilmaz *et al*, 1999), and in the diagnosis of peripheral vascular disease (Joyce *et al*, 1990; Couse *et al*, 1994; Jawahar *et al*, 1997: Johansson *et al*, 2002).

Mode of action

The mode of action of the pulse oximeter is based on Lambert Beer's Law. The law defines the correlation between light transmission and optical density, relating the concentration of a solute to the intensity of light transmitted through it (Ridlen, 1998). The pulse oximeter measures the oxygen saturation of haemoglobin in blood or tissue. The device passes light at two different frequencies — visible red (660 nm) and infrared (900 nm) — through a sensor to a photodetector.

Sensors are available as either transmission or reflectance models. Transmission models have separate light sources and photodetectors, and measure light passing through the subject (eg. digit or earlobe). Reflectance probes have the light source and photodetector mounted in the same probe. These are used over bony areas, such as the anterior tibia, and measure reflected light. For measurement of LOI, the transmission models are more appropriate. The amount of oxygenated haemoglobin (which absorbs more infrared light), and deoxygenated haemoglobin (which absorbs more red light) are measured (Ahrens and Tucker, 1999). The ratio of red to infrared light absorbed determines the oxygen saturation detected by the pulse oximeter. More importantly, pulse oximetry — like Doppler — depends on the presence of pulsatile blood flow, therefore, occlusion of the arteries by a pressure cuff will result in signal loss.

Development of the Lanarkshire Oximetry Index

Arterial screening by pulse oximetry Lanarkshire Oximetry Index (LOI) was developed as a vascular assessment tool for leg ulcer patients. The technique involves simply placing the transducer on a digit which may make it less dependent on operator technique than Doppler ABPI. The following section outlines a protocol to determine suitability for compression therapy.

The Lanarkshire Oximetry Index

Explain the procedure to the patient. Ensure he/she is lying comfortably in a semi-recumbent position.

Stage 1
Measurement of finger oximetry pressure

- An appropriately sized blood-pressure cuff is placed around the upper arm.

- The pulse oximetry sensor is placed on any finger (*Figure 3.1*). When the sensor is placed on the digit, the oximetry will display two numbers; the first represents the patient's heart rate, the second the percentage of circulating oxygenated haemoglobin (SpO_2). Pulsatile blood flow is also displayed either by waveform or a column of lights. A baseline pulse oximetry reading is recorded.

- The sphygmomanometer cuff is inflated to 60 mmHg, then inflated in 10 mmHg increments with approximately 10 seconds between incremental changes. Once the pressure measured reaches 100 mmHg, incremental changes can be increased to 20 mmHg.

- When the pulse oximetry signal is lost (loss of signal is indicated by flattening of the waveform or loss of the column of lights on the oximeter), the pressure reading one below is recorded, eg. if the signal is lost at 180 mmHg, a pressure of 160 mmHg is noted.

- If 180 mmHg is reached before loss of signal, the cuff is not inflated further and a maximum pressure of 180 mmHg is recorded.

- The measurement is repeated on the other arm and the higher of the two readings is used to calculate the LOI.

Measurement of toe oximetry pressure

- An appropriately sized cuff is placed around the ankle immediately above the malleoli. It is important that any fragile skin or ulcer tissue is protected beforehand.

- The oximetry sensor is placed on one of the first three toes (*Figure 3.2*).

- The cuff is inflated as outlined (stage 1) and the pressure at which the signal is lost, or 180 mmHg, if this is reached without loss of signal, is recorded.

Stage 2
Calculate toe/finger oximetry index (ratio)

- The LOI for each leg is calculated by dividing toe pressure by finger pressure and expressing it as a decimal. For example:

> Toe pressure = 140 mmHg
> Finger pressure = 120 mmHg
> LOI = toe pressure/finger pressure = 140/120 = 1.17

Values are similar to those of Doppler ABPI. Patients with a ratio of 0.8 or above can have full compression applied.

Stage 3

- Apply an appropriate graduated compression bandage or stocking to the leg and then place the sensor on one of the first three toes (*Figure 3.3*). The signal is checked with the leg horizontal, then elevated for approximately 30 seconds.

The pulse oximetry test is carried out with patients in a semi-recumbent position, not supine as recommended for Doppler ABPI. Clinical experience shows that many elderly patients with comorbidities affecting their cardiovascular or respiratory systems find lying flat particularly uncomfortable. Thus, pulse oximetry testing may be beneficial in this patient group.

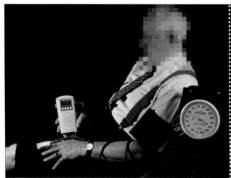

Figure 3.1: Assessing the arm pressure using pulse oximetry

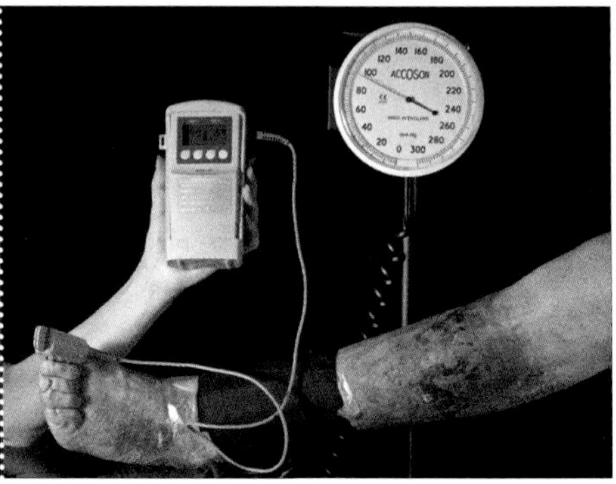

Figure 3.2: Assessing the maximum compression pressure of the toe using pulse oximetry in increments until the signal disappears

In a pilot study, the test was evaluated and Lucke *et al* (1999) demonstrated, by satisfactory healing rates and the absence of bandage damage, that compression could be safely applied to a group of patients with reduced Doppler ABPI, but occlusion pressures of more than 80 mmHg. Subsequently, Bianchi *et al* (2000) found that there was no difference in healing rates in 77 venous ulcer patients selected for suitability for compression by pulse oximetry, irrespective

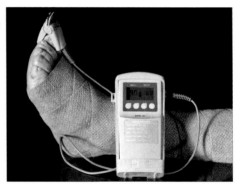

Figure 3.3: Once the compression bandage is in place, the pulse oximeter can be placed on the toe to check for a pulse signal

of whether Doppler ABPI and LOI with a weighted kappa of 0.39. The study found no evidence of ischaemia in patients where toe pulse oximetry reading was normal; however, the sample size used was small so needs interpreting with caution.

In a further study by Zamiri *et al* (2004), 108 patients (200 legs) had ABPI and LOI measurements recorded. The results indicated a fair agreement between the two tests (weighted kappa = 0.484). Of the 200 legs assessed, neither ABPI or LOI could be recorded in one case, and in nine, LOI was recordable but ABPI was not. A Bland-Altman plot indicated neither LOI or ABPI consistently over- or under-read compared to the average of both values, ie. that neither is clearly a better measure than the other. The authors suggested that pulse oximetry LOI was a simple alternative to Doppler ABPI. Further studies comparing pulse oximetry LOI to angiography are currently being undertaken.

Limitations of LOI vascular assessment

The pulse oximetry signal may be difficult to detect if the patient has grossly dystrophic toenails, extreme cyanosis, or, in conditions where there is peripheral vasoconstriction, such as Raynaud's disease. Additionally, LOI will not detect localised arterial disease where there is adequate collateral circulation. If it is necessary to assess blood flow to individual arteries, Doppler ABPI should be used.

These limitations apply to a small percentage of patients but should be considered when carrying out vascular assessment using pulse oximetry.

Conclusion

Studies have suggested that pulse oximetry LOI is at least as effective as Doppler ABPI in the vascular assessment of leg ulcer patients. It may offer advantages in that the instrument is widely available, appears to be simple to use and is less operator-dependent than Doppler. Additionally, the signal can be picked up easily in situations where Doppler ABPI can be problematic, such as in patients with oedema/lymphoedema.

Our own experience and the current literature suggest that where Doppler is used on a regular basis, there may be little need for an additional vascular assessment tool. However, where there is technical difficulty with locating arteries with Doppler ABPI, or where vascular assessment is carried out less frequently, pulse oximetry LOI may provide a suitable, yet simpler, alternative.

References

Ahrens T, Tucker K (1999) Pulse oximetry. *Crit Care Nurs Clin N Am* **11**(1): 87–98

Bianchi J, Douglas WS (2002) Pulse oximetry vascular assessment in leg ulcer patients. *Br J Community Nurs* **7**(9)(suppl): 22–8

Bianchi J, Douglas S, Dawe RS, *et al* (2000) Pulse oximetry: a new tool to assess patients with leg ulcers. *J Wound Care* **9**(3): 109–12

Callam MJ, Ruckley CV, Dale JJ, Harper DR (1987a) Hazards of compression treatment of the leg: an estimate from Scottish surgeons. *Br Med J* **295**: 1382

Callam MJ, Harper DR, Dale JJ, Ruckley CV (1987b) Arterial disease in chronic leg ulceration: an underestimated hazard? Lothian and Forth Valley leg ulcer study. *Br J Med* **294**: 929–31

Clinical Resource Efficiency Support Team (CREST) (1998) *Guidelines for the Assessment and Management of Leg Ulcers.* CREST, Belfast

Couse NF, Delaney CP, Horgan PG, *et al* (1994) Pulse oximetry in the diagnosis of non-critical peripheral vascular disease. *J Roy Soc Med* **87**(9): 511–12

Cullum N, Nelson EA, Fletcher AW, Sheldon TA (2002) *Compression for venous leg ulcers* (Cochrane Review). In: The Cochrane Library, issue 2. Update Software, Oxford

Eichorn JH, Cooper JB, Cullen DJ, Maier WR, Philip JH, Seeman RG (1986) Standards of patient monitoring during anaesthesia at Harvard Medical School. *J Am Acad Med* **256**: 1017–20

Fletcher A, Cullum N, Sheldon TA (1997) A systematic review of compression treatment for venous leg ulcers. *Br Med J* **315**: 576–80

Fowkes FGR, Housley E, MacIntyre CCA, Prescott RJ, Ruckley CV (1988) Variability of ankle brachial systolic pressures in the measurement of artherosclerotic peripheral arteries. *J Epidemiol Comm Health* **42**(2): 128–33

Jawahar D, Rachamalla HR, Rafalowski A, Ilkani R, Bharathan T, Anandarao N (1997) Pulse oximetry in the evaluation of peripheral vascular disease. *Angiology* **48**(8): 721–4

Johaansson KEA, Marklund BRG, Fowelin JHR (2002) Evaluation of a new screening method for detecting peripheral arterial disease in a primary health care population of patients with diabetes mellitus. *Diabetic Med* **19**: 307–10

Joyce WP, Walsh K, Gough DB, Gorey TF, Fitzpatrick JM (1990) Pulse oximetry: a new non-invasive assessment of peripheral arterial occlusive disease. *Br J Surg* **77**(10): 1115–17

Kaiser V, Kester ADM, Stoffers HE (1999) The influence of experience on the reproducibility of the ankle-brachial systolic pressure ratio in peripheral arterial occlusive disease. _Eur J Vasc Endovasc Surg_ **18**: 25–9

Lindsay LA, Watson JD, Quaba AA (1991) Pulse oximetry in monitoring of free muscle flaps. _Br J Plastic Surg_ **44**: 27–9

Lucke TW, Urcelay M, Bianchi J, Loney M, McEvoy M, Douglas WS (1999) Pulse oximetry: an additional tool in the assessment of patients with leg ulcers. _Br J Dermatol_ **141**(Suppl 55): 65

Millikan GA (1942) The oximeter, an instrument for measuring continuously the oxygen saturation of arterial blood in man. _Rev Sci Instruments_ **13**: 434–4

Modi KD, Sharma AK, Mishra SK, Mithal A (1997) Pulse oximetry for the assessment of autonomic neuropathy in diabetic patients. _J Diabetes Complications_ **11**: 35–9

Ray SA, Srodon PD, Taylor RS, Dormandy JA (1994) Reliability of ankle: brachial pressure index measurement by junior doctors. _Br J Surg_ **81**: 188–90

Ridlen G (1998) Pulse oximetry: a historical perspective. _J Resp Care Practitioners_ **11**(5): 47–50

Royal College of Nursing (1998) _The Management of Patients with Venous Leg Ulcers_. RCN, York

Scottish Intercollegiate Guidelines Network (1998) _The Care of Patients with Chronic Leg Ulcers_. SIGN, Edinburgh

Severinghaus JW, Astrup PB, Murray JF (1998) Blood gas analysis and critical care medicine. _Am J Resp Crit Care Med_ **4**(Suppl): 114–22

Squire JR (1940) Instrument for measuring quality of blood and its degree of oxygenation in web of the hand. _Clin Sci_ **4**: 331–9

Stephen CR, Slater HM, Johnson AL, Sekelj P (1951) The oximeter – a technical aid for the anaesthesiologist. _Anaesthesiology_ **12**: 541–5

Strandness DE, Schultz RD, Sumner DS, Rushmer RF (1967) Ultrasonic flow detection: A useful technique in the evaluation of peripheral vascular disease. _Am J Surg_ **113**: 311–20

Tremper KK, Barker SJ (1989) Pulse oximetry. _Anesthesiology_ **70**: 98–108

Vowden KR, Vowden P (2002) Can the cuff position be varied when recording ABPI? _J Wound Care_ **11**(7): 250

Wood EH, Geraci JE (1949) Photoelectric determination of arterial saturation in man. _J Lab Clin Med_ **34**: 387–401

Woodrow P (1999) Pulse oximetry. _Nurs Standard_ **13**(42): 42–6

Yilmaz EN, Vahl AC, van Rij G, Nauta SH, Brom HL, Rauwerda JA (1999) Endoluminal pulse oximetry of the sigmoid colon and the monitoring of colonic circulation. _Cardiovasc Surg_ **7**(7): 704–9

Zamiri M, Bianchi J, Loney M, Dawe RS, Douglas WS (2004) Pulse oximetry: A simpler method of arterial assessment in venous dermatitis and leg ulcer. *J Am Acad Dermatol* **50**(S1): 168

CHAPTER 4

BEST PRACTICE FOR TREATING AND MANAGING PRESSURE ULCERS

Pam Cooper and David Gray

NHS Quality Improvement Scotland (NHS QIS) was set up by the Scottish Parliament in 2003 to take the lead in improving the quality of care and treatment delivered by NHS Scotland. The purpose of NHS QIS is to improve the quality of health care in Scotland by setting standards and monitoring performance, and by providing NHS Scotland with advice, guidance and support on effective clinical practice and service improvements.

This chapter will present the Best Practice Statement for the Treatment/Management of Pressure Ulcers which was launched in May 2005. These statements reflect current best practice within a recognised specialist group of practitioners, along with best graded evidence available. Best practice statements (BPSs) are designed to reflect the slight variances in care across the multiple care settings but, in doing so, ensuring that everybody is attaining a certain baseline standardisation in their care to ensure best outcomes for their patients. The chapter is a direct translation of the statement to enhance care in the treatment/management of pressure ulcers across all care settings.

Best practice statements

While many examples of clinical guidelines exist there is a lack of reliable statements focusing specifically on nursing and midwifery practice. The development of BPSs reflects the current emphasis on delivering care that is patient-centred, cost-effective and fair, and is an attempt to reduce existing variations in practice. Following the full implementation of BPSs, it is hoped that there will be comparable standards of care for patients wherever they access services.

What is a best practice statement?

BPSs describe best and achievable practice in a specific area of care. The use of the term 'best practice' reflects the NHS QIS's commitment to sharing local excellence at national level. BPSs are underpinned by a number of key principles (*Table 4.1*).

Table 4.1: The key principles of best practice statements
Best practice statements are intended to guide practice and promote a consistent and cohesive approach to care
Best practice statements are primarily intended for use by registered nurses, midwives and the staff who support them, but they may also contribute to multidisciplinary working, and be of guidance to other members of the healthcare team
Statements are derived from the best available evidence at the time they are produced, recognising that levels and types of evidence vary
Information is gathered from a broad range of sources in order to identify existing or previous initiatives at local and national level, incorporate work of a qualitative and quantitative nature and establish consensus
Statements are targeted at practitioners, using language that is accessible and meaningful
Consultation with relevant organisations and individuals is undertaken
Statements will be nationally reviewed and updated, if necessary, every three years
Responsibility for implementation of statements will rest at local level
Key sources of evidence and available resources are provided

Use of evidence in best practice statements

The need to embrace evidence in its broadest sense has been acknowledged by NHS QIS in the development of its BPSs. The statements represent a unique synthesis of evidence derived from research, audit, patient surveys, expert opinion, professional consensus and patient/public experience. In developing the statements a rigorous, transparent and consistent 'bottom-up' approach is adopted to articulate best practice that involves professionals and patients and which is based on all types of available evidence. The following stages describe the process of identifying and reviewing evidence for inclusion in statements:

- define question
- review evidence from a range of sources, including published literature, grey literature (information sheets, magazines, etc) and other relevant sources, eg. patient groups, manufacturers and professional groups
- integrate evidence with patient-related factors, eg. issues of access, equity and ethics
- develop recommendations
- evaluate process and impact of recommendations.

The key stages in the development of BPSs are shown in *Figure 4.1.*

Selection of topics

In order to identify the priorities for the development of BPSs, an extensive consultation process is undertaken involving the practice development unit's link nurse/midwife network, the Directors of Nursing Group and other organisations. The following criteria guide the choice of topics:

- the selection of areas of broad significance to nursing/midwifery as a whole rather than being specialty specific. This may facilitate cross-boundary working between specialties, promote greater uptake of statements and have a wider impact on patient care
- the identification of areas where there is evidence of variation in practice affecting patient care
- the use of research recommendations to identify topics for the development of statements
- a focus on practice issues rather than service provision.

How the statement should be used

The BPS has a variety of uses, although primarily it is intended to promote evidence-based practice. Each statement aims to be realistic but challenging and can be used:

- as a basis for developing and improving care
- to stimulate learning among teams
- to promote effective interdisciplinary team-working

- to determine whether a quality service is being provided
- to stimulate ideas and priorities for nursing research
- as an educational tool for pre- and post-registration students.

A working group was established to review the document at various draft versions to ensure that information obtained reflected best practice. This working group consisted of tissue viability nurses from across Scotland.

Best Practice Statement on Treatment/ Management of Pressure Ulcers

Pressure ulcers are areas of tissue death usually located over a bony prominence, and are caused by external forces of pressure, shear and/ or friction. This situation may be further exacerbated by complications arising from the individual's physical condition, such as altered nutrition and excess moisture.

The treatment/management of pressure ulcers is often fraught, as there are a vast array of interventions available, ranging from pressure-reducing surfaces to the physical treatment of the wound itself. This has led to confusion among practitioners, with little consensus about good practice across the multiple care settings. The Best Practice Statement for the Treatment/Management of Pressure Ulcers has therefore been produced by NHS QIS to offer guidance to nurses, midwives, health visitors, untrained nursing staff and carers, who look after individuals with existing pressure ulcers within hospitals, homes or care homes. It aims to provide staff, patients and carers with a framework that can be utilised when making decisions relating to the treatment/management of pressure ulcers. The statement does not give specific details relating to product selection, as it is intended to be used in conjunction with local policies and guidelines.

The BPS should be used in conjunction with the Best Practice Statement for the Prevention of Pressure Ulcers (www.nhshealthquality. org). Utilisation of both documents will ensure that best practice is being achieved across all care settings. All tissue viability nurses within Scotland have been involved in the development of these documents.

The implementation of this BPS will represent a challenge to all healthcare providers. Those organisations that employ tissue viability specialists will be able to use them as a source of advice on strategies for implementation. Other organisations will have to consider

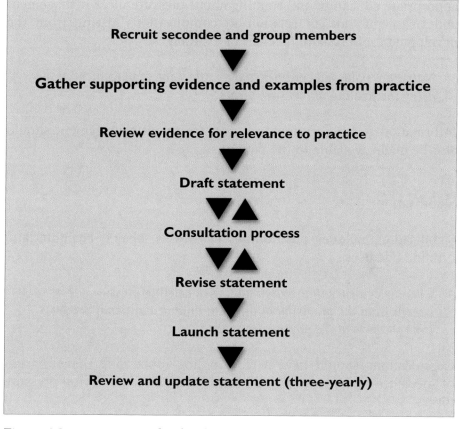

Figure 4.1: Key stages in the development of best practice statements

implementation strategies that best suit local needs. The BPS covers three main areas: assessment, stabilisation, and treatment.

Assessment of the individual

Assessment comprises classification, pressure ulcer assessment, history, physical examination, and exacerbating complications, eg. nutrition, pain, continence:

> *The underlying principle is that all patients with pressure ulcers have their ulcers classified and assessed in conjunction with their overall physical condition.*

Staff and carers looking after individuals with pressure ulcers need appropriate education and training about pressure ulcer management and treatment, and in relation to complications arising from the development of pressure ulcers. For example:

Nutrition, pain and continence may affect the management of, or delay the healing of pressure ulcers.

Information relating to pressure ulcer treatment/management should also be made available to the patient.

Stabilisation

Stabilisation includes positioning, mattresses, chairs, cushions and orthodox devices:

There is evidence that individuals with existing pressure ulcers benefit from the provision of different and/or additional products from the standard equipment provided.

Organisations should have a clear policy concerning the provision of specialist equipment for individuals recognised as having pressure ulcers.

Treatment

Treatment involves promoting healing (such as wound cleansing), debridement, and managing bacterial colonisation and infection:

The treatment of pressure ulcers should follow the principles of moist wound healing, with removal of devitalised tissue, the appropriate treatment of infection and stimulation of wound healing.

Health records should show evidence of a clear plan of care for the management and treatment of the pressure ulcer, with regular review and evidence of assessment.

Each section of the BPS contains a table corresponding to the what, why and how of best practice, ie. detail of what is to be achieved, the reason for this and how to achieve it, or to demonstrate it is being achieved. In addition, each section identifies key points and/or challenges for primary care or care home settings and further tables and/or appendices about specific points.

Definition and classification

Pressure ulcers are areas of localised damage to the skin and underlying tissue, as a result of occlusion of the blood vessels which leads to cell death. They are believed to be caused by pressure, shear and friction (Allman, 1997; European Pressure Ulcer Advisory Panel (EPUAP), 1999). A pressure ulcer classification system is as follows:

- *Grade 1:* non-blanchable erythema of intact skin. Discoloration of the skin, warmth, oedema, induration or hardness may also be used as indicators, particularly on individuals with darker skin.
- *Grade 2:* partial-thickness skin loss involving epidermis, dermis, or both. The ulcer is superficial and presents clinically as an abrasion or blister.
- *Grade 3:* full-thickness skin loss involving damage to, or necrosis of subcutaneous tissue that may extend down to, but not through, underlying fascia.
- *Grade 4:* extensive destruction, tissue necrosis, or damage to muscle, bone or supporting structures with or without full-thickness skin loss (EPUAP, 1999).

Grade 1 and 2 pressure ulcers are described as superficial within this BPS, while grade 3 and 4 pressure ulcers are defined as severe.

Section 1: Assessment/classification

❖ All individuals with pressure ulcers should have the ulcers assessed using a recognised grading scale.
❖ Staff involved in assessing the pressure ulcer(s) should receive training and regular updates.

Statement

1. All individuals identified with existing pressure ulcers have their ulcer(s) assessed to determine level of tissue damage, using a

recognised classification tool such as EPUAP (1999), Stirling (Reid and Morrison, 1994), Pressure Ulcer Scale for Healing (PUSH) (Stotts *et al*, 2001).
2. The pressure ulcer(s) should be reassessed regularly, at least weekly, or according to the individual's condition and/or if the individual's condition changes.
3. Staff involved in assessing pressure ulcer(s) receive training and regular update sessions on pressure ulcer classification and treatment.

Reasons for statement

1. Grading of pressure ulcer damage enables correct and suitable treatment and intervention to be initiated and maintained.
2. Most pressure ulcers observed within Scotland are of a superficial nature (Gray *et al*, 1999; Watret, 1999).
3. Assessment and reassessment allow for an accurate and individualised treatment plan to be devised.

How to demonstrate statement is being achieved

1. The health records of all individuals identified as having an existing pressure ulcer(s) include evidence of pressure ulcer grading, from initial onset.
2. There is documented evidence that all individuals with existing pressure ulcers receive treatment and interventions appropriate to their condition.
3. There is documented evidence that the individual's condition and pressure ulcer are reassessed regularly, at least weekly, or more frequently according to the individual's condition.
4. Records of staff training in assessment and treatment are available.

Section 2: Assessment

❖ Treatment of pressure ulcers can only commence once a full assessment of the ulcer has been carried out.

Statement

1. The pressure ulcer is assessed initially for cause, location, grade,

dimensions, wound bed appearance, exudate, pain, surrounding skin condition and critical colonisation/infection.
2. Pressure ulcer(s) are reassessed at least weekly, or more frequently, according to the individual's condition.

Reasons for statement

1. Early identification of skin changes (*Appendix 4.1*) and/or thorough assessment of the pressure ulcer(s) are needed to inform appropriate treatments and interventions. Thorough assessment allows for the identification of underlying tissue involvement as well as sinus formation.
2. Early identification and treatment of underlying tissue involvement and/or sinus formation reduce the risk of complications and enable appropriate rationale and associated treatment interventions to be determined.
3. Evidence suggests that treatment can only commence once a full assessment of the pressure ulcer has been achieved.
4. The pressure ulcer(s) requires reassessment to observe alteration in pressure ulcer condition.

How to demonstrate statement is being achieved

1. The health records of all individuals identified with a graded pressure ulcer include documented evidence of pressure ulcer wound assessment and any interventions carried out or adopted.
2. There is documented evidence that staff act on individual components identified while assessing the wound or individual.
3. Health records show evidence of assessment and a rationale for treatment aims and objectives.
4. The health records contain evidence of reassessment of pressure ulcers where possible, at least weekly, or according to the individual's condition.

Section 3: History and physical condition

❖ Deterioration in the pressure ulcer or the individual's physical condition are closely related and the two should be assessed together.

Statement

1. A complete history and physical examination of the individual is undertaken.
2. If the condition of the individual or of the wound deteriorates, the situation is re-evaluated and a new or updated treatment rationale and plan identified.

Reasons for statement

1. A pressure ulcer should be assessed in the context of the individual's overall physical and psychosocial health.
2. Deterioration in either the individual's physical condition or pressure ulcer(s) are closely related and, therefore, should be assessed together.

How to demonstrate statement is being achieved

1. There is evidence within the individual's health records that staff act on individual components identified through history and physical examination.
2. Identified deterioration in either the individual's physical condition or pressure ulcer(s) is recorded in the health record along with any subsequent action taken.

Section 4: Complications

❖ Adequate dietary intake for individuals with pressure ulcers must be ensured.
❖ Pressure ulcers can be painful and treatment may increase the pain.

Statement

1. Adequate dietary intake for individuals with evidence of pressure ulcer(s) is ensured.
2. Individuals with altered nutritional status have their intake of food and fluid reassessed regularly.
3. The individual's overall psychosocial health is assessed to determine causes of pain.
4. The advice of specialist(s) is sought if necessary.

5. Pain related to the pressure ulcer(s) or their treatment is assessed and appropriate interventions undertaken.

Reasons for statement

1. Evidence suggests that individuals who are malnourished may have delayed or altered healing rates as a result of the lack of calorific value of their diet (Clark *et al*, 2004; Mathus-Vliegen, 2004).
2. Regular assessment of intake enables timely interventions.
3. Treatment interventions may affect pain levels, in some cases increasing the pain.
4. Pain may occur as a result of the presence of pressure ulcers (Reddy *et al*, 2003).

How to demonstrate statement is being achieved

1. The health records of all individuals with altered nutritional intake include evidence of assessment and/or interventions.
2. The result of nutritional review and any changes made are documented.
3. The advice of a dietitian is sought where dietary review and supplements may be indicated.
4. The health record documents measures to eliminate or control the source of pain by appropriate interventions, eg. covering wound, adjusting support surfaces, repositioning and analgesia if required.
5. Health records include an indication of interventions taken in response to pain.
6. There is evidence that staff act on individual aspects of the causes of pain.
7. Evidence of medication or other methods of pain relief are recorded along with outcome measures.

Section 5: Continence

* Incontinence can increase the risk of pressure ulcer development.
* Cleansing with soap and water can contribute to the development of pressure ulcers.
* Barrier creams should not be used with superficial pressure ulcers.

Statement

1. Individuals with incontinence have their continence status reassessed regularly or according to the individual's condition.
2. Continence management should be reviewed regularly.
3. Soap and water should not be used when cleansing following episodes of incontinence.
4. Products which promote a moist wound environment are used unless contraindicated by the individual's condition.
5. For individuals with superficial pressure ulcers (broken skin) as a result of incontinence, refer to the section on 'Promoting healing'.

Reasons for statement

1. Incontinence can increase an individual's risk of pressure ulcer development as a result of chemical irritation and/or the inappropriate cleansing regime adopted (Cooper and Gray, 2001).
2. Changes in continence (incontinence pattern, cleansing regime used) can contribute to the development of pressure ulcers.
3. Cleansing with soap and water can contribute to the development of pressure ulcers (Cooper and Gray, 2001).
4. Barrier creams have no role to play in skin care for superficial pressure ulcers of intact or broken skin; superficial pressure ulcers (broken skin) should be managed by moist wound healing (please refer to the section on 'Promoting healing').

How to demonstrate statement is being achieved

1. Health records include evidence that regular skin inspection takes place at opportune times, eg. during assistance with personal hygiene.
2. Findings from skin inspection indicating that further action is required, along with subsequent action taken, are recorded in the patient's health record.
3. The health records document episodes of incontinence and indicate action taken, including skin cleansing products used.
4. The advice of a continence adviser is sought where continence management products are compromised by pressure ulcer treatment strategies.
5. The health records contain evidence of ongoing assessment, treatment rationale and interventions taken.

Section 6: Stabilisation — positioning

❖ Individuals with pressure ulcers must not be cared for on a standard NHS mattress or on a basic divan.
❖ Delay in the provision of pressure-reducing equipment may result in further tissue damage.
❖ Regular skin inspection and any subsequent action taken are documented in health records.

Statement

1. Individuals with a pressure ulcer(s) are suitably positioned to minimise pressure, friction, shear and the potential for further tissue damage.
2. Individuals who can move independently are encouraged/enabled to do so.
3. Individuals who require assistance with movement are educated, along with associated carers, in the benefits and techniques of weight distribution.
4. Individuals with specific moving and handling requirements (ie. spinal injuries) have their needs assessed by those with relevant skills and in relation to their whole physical condition.

Reasons for statement

1. Pressure is the main factor in the development of pressure ulcers; friction and shear can also play a part in their development.
2. The time span between position changes is dependent on individual assessment. Individuals with a pressure ulcer should not be positioned in a seat for more than two hours without some form of repositioning (DeFloor and Grypdonck, 1999). NB. In the community setting this can only be advised.
3. Devices to assist with the repositioning of individuals in bed, ie. profiling beds, electric and non-electric bed frames, are of value.
4. Moving and handling aids such as hoists and slings can also be used to reposition the individual.

How to demonstrate statement is being achieved

1. Health records include an indication of how frequently position changes are to be carried out.

2. Records indicate that:
   - individuals with a pressure ulcer are not positioned in a seat for more than two hours, without being repositioned; acutely ill patients are returned to bed for no less than one hour (Gebhardt and Bliss, 1994; Defloor and Grypdonck, 1999)
   - when possible, the individual and/or carer are involved in the management of weight distribution of individuals who are wheelchair dependent (please refer to Best Practice Statement for the Prevention of Pressure Ulcers)
   - for individuals in bed, differing positions such as the 30-degree tilt are used (Young, 2004). The 30-degree tilt is when the patient is placed in the laterally inclined position, supported by pillows, with his or her back making a 30-degree angle with the support surface
   - hoist slings and sliding sheets are not left under individuals after use (where there are associated manual handling issues concerning the removal of a hoist sling, a joint assessment by tissue viability/manual handling advisers should be documented)
   - skin inspection, at least weekly, is carried out after each positional change; these inspections help to guide decisions on the length of time between positional changes.
3. Independent movement is encouraged and patient education is documented in the health records.
4. The result of skin inspection and any changes made to the repositioning regime are documented.
5. Health records show evidence of referral to physiotherapist and/or occupational therapist to assist with mobility or position changing where appropriate.

Section 7: Stabilisation — mattresses, chairs and cushions

Statement

1. Individuals with a pressure ulcer(s) are not cared for on standard NHS mattresses or on basic divan mattresses; as a minimum they are provided with a pressure-reducing foam mattress or overlay. (A standard NHS mattress is classified as: a standard foam mattress, block or cut foam, but which is not classified as

a pressure-reducing mattress.) Factors taken into account when deciding on which pressure-reducing equipment to purchase or hire include: clinical efficacy; ease of maintenance; impact on care procedures; patient acceptability; cost; and ease of use.

2. The decision to provide any pressure-reducing equipment is taken as part of a comprehensive treatment/management strategy, never as a sole intervention.

3. Individuals being cared for on specialist equipment have their skin inspected frequently to assess the suitability of the equipment; equipment requirements may change with alterations in the patient's condition.

4. Individuals with pressure ulcers are provided with appropriate pressure-reducing equipment when sitting in a chair or wheelchair, in addition to when they are being cared for in bed.

5. Long-term wheelchair or static seat users have their needs assessed by those with relevant specialist skills.

Reasons for statement

1. There is clear evidence that individuals with pressure ulcers benefit from the provision of different/additional products from the standard NHS issue (Cullum *et al*, 2000; McInnes and National Institute for Clinical Excellence[NICE], 2004).

2. Individuals with an existing pressure ulcer who are acutely ill or who have restricted mobility in bed are likely to require an air-filled mattress or overlay.

3. There is no clear evidence as to the best products to use (McInnes and National Institute for Clinical Excellence, 2004).

4. Individuals identified as requiring pressure-reducing equipment (mattresses, seating, and cushions) should receive it as soon as possible as delay may result in further tissue damage occurring (Best Practice Statement for the Prevention of Pressure Ulcers).

5. Further tissue damage may occur when patients are sitting in chairs (Defloor and Grypdonck, 1999).

6. Chairs and/or cushions designed to reduce the risk of pressure ulcer development must be suited to individual needs in relation to the individual's height, weight, postural alignment and foot support.

7. The safety of static seats can be compromised as a result of changes in height, balance and lumbar support with the use of cushions (Collins, 2000).

8. People have individual requirements based on their overall condition and skin condition and their own previous experience.

How to demonstrate statement is being achieved

1. There is a clear organisational policy concerning the provision of specialist equipment for individuals with existing pressure ulcers; the policy includes guidance of when to seek advice from a tissue viability specialist.
2. The decision to use any product beyond a basic NHS mattress or divan is documented in the individual's health record.
3. Measures being implemented (ie. positional changes), in addition to the use of special mattresses and overlays, are documented in the health record.
4. The date of first use of specialist equipment is documented in the health record.
5. Regular skin inspection, at least weekly or according to the individual's condition, and any subsequent actions taken/ decisions made, are documented in the health record.
6. The individual's health record documents the assessment of his or her needs in relation to his or her wheelchair/static seat use.

Section 8: Promoting healing

Statement

1. Extensive superficial pressure ulcers (5% of body) or any severe pressure ulcers should be considered for referral to a specialist service, such as tissue viability or plastic surgery.
2. Each individual with a pressure ulcer has a clear plan of management outlined in his/her health record.
3. The management of the wound bed of a pressure ulcer adheres to the principles of moist wound management unless the individual's condition dictates otherwise.

Reasons for statement

1. The management of individuals with large areas of superficial ulcers or severe ulcers requires specialist input because of the potential for the development of life-threatening complications (ie. septicaemia).

2. Pressure ulcers are likely to require a number of weeks or months to heal depending on their severity and the individual's co-morbidity.
3. Wounds that are managed using products which promote moist wound healing result in enhanced healing rates and reduced infection rates.

How to demonstrate statement is being achieved

1. Health records show that individuals with extensive superficial pressure ulceration are referred for a specialist review unless the individual's condition dictates otherwise.
2. Health records show that individuals with severe pressure ulceration are referred for a specialist review unless the individual's condition dictates otherwise.
3. The health records of the individual referred for specialist review reflect the nature of referral, eg. telephone or letter, and the outcome of the referral, eg. telephone advice or direct consultation.
4. Health records include evidence that individuals with a pressure ulcer(s) have a full assessment of the ulcer(s) and their management plan is documented; this incorporates steps taken to ensure continuity between different care settings.
5. The health record includes all formal referrals or informal discussions with specialists regarding the management of the individual.
6. Evidence of initial and ongoing management to prevent further tissue damage should be evident.

Section 9: Wound cleansing

Statement

1. Wounds are cleansed to remove visible debris and to aid assessment.
2. Excess loose slough and exudate is removed before assessment and/or dressing change.
3. Wounds are cleansed with warm tap water, or warm saline; irrigation of the wound or showering is recommended (Miller and Glover, 1996).

Reasons for statement

1. Wound cleansing is advised to remove excess exudate, slough or debris to aid wound assessment, but does not remove bacteria present (Rodeheaver, 1999).
2. Removal of excess loose slough and exudate will remove any associated odour, and will also permit a more accurate assessment of the wound (Romanelli and Mastronicola, 2002).

How to demonstrate statement is being achieved

1. The health records of individuals who require their wound to be cleansed include cleansing method used.
2. There is evidence that pressure ulcers with excess exudate, slough or debris are cleansed.
3. There are clear local policies for wound cleansing.
4. There is evidence that staff select and document the appropriate method of cleansing to best meet the needs of the individual and his/her wound.

Section 10: Debridement

❖ The presence of devitalised tissue delays the healing process.

Statement

1. Devitalised tissue in pressure ulcer(s) is removed where appropriate for the individual's condition and in conjunction with the individual goals.
2. Superficial (broken skin) pressure ulcers may benefit from autolytic debridement techniques.
3. Severe pressure ulcers may benefit from sharp, autolytic and biosurgery debridement techniques where appropriate
4. For individuals who are terminally ill or with other co-morbidities, overall quality of life should be considered before deciding whether and how to debride.
5. For spreading cellulitis or sepsis, sharp debridement can be used where appropriate (please refer to 'Managing bacterial colonisation and infection', *p. 47*).

Reasons for statement

1. The presence of devitalised tissue delays the healing process by keeping the wound in the inflammatory phase of wound healing; removal of devitalised tissue helps prevent the spread of infection (Romanelli and Mastronicola, 2002).
2. Local infection can be managed using antimicrobial wound management products.

How to demonstrate statement is being achieved

1. Records indicate that the individual's condition has been assessed before any decision is taken to remove devitalised tissue, as well as demonstrating the rationale for product choice and a clear process for review.
2. Sharp debridement can be used where appropriate by a person considered competent to do so (usually a nurse, surgeon or podiatrist).
3. Modern wound management products can facilitate the removal of devitalised tissue and products selected are recorded in the health records.
4. Health records demonstrate that assessment of the local infection has been undertaken, action taken and review planned.

Section 11: Managing bacterial colonisation and infection

❖ All pressure ulcers are colonised with bacteria.
❖ Most local infection can be managed using topical antimicrobial products.
❖ Systemic antibiotics should not be used routinely for local infection.
❖ Assessment and regular review of local infection are documented.

Statement

1. The risk of infection in individuals with existing pressure ulcers is reduced.
2. Where there is devitalised tissue present, its removal is facilitated by using debridement techniques, unless the individual's overall condition contraindicates debridement.

3. Routine wound swabs are not required unless clinically indicated, according to local infection control policies.
4. Systemic antibiotics are not to be used as a matter of routine where local infection is present, although are indicated for particular conditions.
5. Infection control guidance is sought when considering the use of topical antibiotics.
6. The advice of an infection control adviser is sought if necessary.

Reasons for statement

1. Avoiding local or spreading infection reduces the risk to the individual of delayed healing, and in extreme cases, death (Cutting and White, 2004).
2. The presence of devitalised tissue in the wound bed can delay healing and increase the risk of infection.
3. Modern wound management products can facilitate the removal of devitalised tissue.
4. All pressure ulcers will be colonised with bacteria and therefore wound swabs should only be taken when clinically indicated, according to local policy.
5. Local infection can be managed using topical antimicrobial wound management products without the use of systemic antibiotics, unless the individual's overall condition dictates otherwise.
6. Spreading infection, bacteraemia, sepsis or osteomyelitis will require the appropriate systemic antibiotic.
7. Evidence suggests that the effects of topical antibiotics are limited and sensitisation commonly occurs.
8. Individuals not responding to systemic antibiotic treatment may require radiological examination to exclude the presence of osteomyelitis or joint infection.

How to demonstrate statement is being achieved

1. All local infection control policies are applied, with particular attention to hand decontamination.
2. Records demonstrate that, where the individual's condition allows, the removal of devitalised tissue has been considered.
3. Records indicate when and why wound swabs have been taken, and the results of the swabs.

4. Health records demonstrate a rationale for product choice and a clear process of review.
5. Health records should demonstrate that assessment of the local infection has been undertaken and that regular reviews are also occurring.
6. Records indicate when and why systemic antibiotics have been prescribed and that advice has also been sought from the microbiology and/or infection control team where required.
7. Health records demonstrate that there is an ongoing assessment of the individual's response to antibiotic treatment.

Conclusion

The Best Practice Statement for the Treatment/Management of Pressure Ulcers was developed through the cooperation, collaboration and consensus of all tissue viability nurses across Scotland. It is hoped that with support it will be accepted and implemented across all clinical settings and organisations. The recent mandatory status of all BPSs within Scotland will give clinicians the support and best evidence available for the management of individuals with pressure ulcers.

References

Allman RM (1997) Pressure ulcer prevalence, incidence, risk factors, and impact. *Clin Geriatr Med* **13**(3): 421–36

Barton A, Barton M (1981) *The Management and Prevention of Pressure Sores*. Faber and Faber, London

Clark M, Defloor T, Bours G (2004) A pilot study of the prevalence of pressure ulcers in European hospitals. In: Clark M, ed. *Pressure Ulcers: Recent Advances in Tissue Viability*. Quay Books, MA Healthcare Ltd, Salisbury: 8–22

Clark M, Schols J, Benati G, *et al* (2004) Pressure ulcers and nutrition: a new European guideline. *J Wound Care* **13**(7): 267–72

Collins F (2000) Selecting the most appropriate armchair for patients. *J Wound Care* **9**(2): 73–6

Cooper P, Gray D (2001) Comparison of two skin care regimes for incontinence. *Br J Nurs* **10**(6; Suppl): S6, S8, S10

Cullum N, Deeks J, Fletcher A, *et al* (1995) The prevention and treatment of pressure ulcers: how useful are the measures for scoring people's risk of developing a pressure sore? *Effective Health Care Bull* 2(1): 1–18 (Available online at: www.york.ac.uk/inst/crd/ehc21.pdf)

Cullum N, Deeks J, Sheldon T, Song F, Fletcher A (2000) Beds, mattresses and cushions for pressure ulcer prevention and treatment. Cochrane Database Syst Rev 2: CD001735. Update in Cochrane Database Syst Rev 2004, 3: CD001735

Defloor T, Grypdonck MH (1999) Sitting posture and prevention of pressure ulcers. *Appl Nurs Res* 12(3): 136–42

European Pressure Ulcer Advisory Panel (1999) Guidelines on treatment of pressure ulcers. *EPUAP Rev* 1(2): 31–3 (www.epuap.org/glprevention. html)

Gebhardt K, Bliss MR (1994) Preventing pressure sores in orthopaedic patients — is prolonged chair nursing detrimental? *J Tissue Viabil* 4(2): 51–4

Gray D, Cooper P, Clark M (1999) *Pressure ulcer prevention in an acute hospital*. Poster presentation, European Pressure Ulcer Advisory Panel (EPUAP), Amsterdam 1999. EPUAP Review

McInnes E, National Institure for Clinical Excellence (2004) The use of pressure-relieving devices (beds, mattresses and overlays) for the prevention of pressure ulcers in primary and secondary care. *J Tissue Viability* 14(1): 4–6, 8, 10 passim

Mathus-Vliegen EM (2004) Old age, malnutrition, and pressure sores: an ill-fated alliance. *J Gerontol Biol Sci Med Sci* 59(4): 355–60

Miller M, Glover D, eds (1999) *Wound Management Theory and Practice*. Nursing Times Books, London

Reddy M, Keast D, Fowler E, Sibbald R (2003) Pain in pressure ulcers. *Ostomy/Wound Management* 49(4 Suppl): 30–5

Reid J, Morrison M (1994) Towards a consensus: classification of pressure sores. *J Wound Care* 3(3): 157–60

Rodeheaver GT (1999) Pressure ulcer debridement and cleansing: a review of current literature. *Ostomy/Wound Management* 45(1A Suppl): 80S–85S

Romanelli M, Mastronicola D (2002) The role of wound-bed preparation in managing chronic pressure ulcers. *J Wound Care* 11(8): 305–10

Stotts NA, Rodeheaver GT, Thomas DR, *et al* (2001) An instrument to measure healing in pressure ulcers: development and validation of the pressure ulcer scale for healing (PUSH). *J Gerontol A Biol Sci Med Sci* 56(12): M795–9

Watret L (1999) Using a case-mix-adjusted pressure sore incidence study in a surgical directorate to improve patient outcomes in pressure ulcer prevention. *J Tissue Viability* 9(4): 121–5

Young T (2004) The 30-degree tilt position vs the 90-degree lateral and supine positions in reducing the incidence of non-blanching erythema in a hospital inpatient population: a randomised controlled trial. *J Tissue Viability* 14(3): 88–96

Appendix 4.1: Further examination of erythema should include the following

Apply light finger pressure to the area for 10 seconds.

Release the pressure. If the area is white and then returns to its original colour, the area probably has an adequate blood supply. Observation should continue and preventative strategies should be employed.

If, on release of pressure, the area remains the same colour as before pressure was applied, it is an indication of the beginning of pressure ulcer development and preventative strategies should be employed.

If there is an alteration in skin colour (redness, purple or black), increased heat or swelling, it may imply underlying tissue breakdown. Frequency of assessment should be increased.

With dark skin pigmentation, pressure ulcer development will be indicated by areas where there is localised heat, or where there is damage, coolness, purple/black discolouration localised oedema and induration.

CHAPTER 5

OPTIMISING NUTRITION TO PREVENT PRESSURE ULCER DEVELOPMENT

Emma Johnston

Pressure ulcers are common in most healthcare settings. Precise estimates of incidence or prevalence are unknown, but figures quoted include prevalence rates of 3–10% and 3–23% depending on the setting (European Pressure Ulcer Advisory Panel [EPUAP], 2002). A pressure ulcer is defined as an 'area of localised damage to the skin and underlying tissue caused by pressure, shear, friction and/or a combination of these' (EPUAP, 1998). Pressure, friction and shear are considered to be extrinsic factors that impinge upon the surface of the skin. In addition, several intrinsic factors can contribute to the development of pressure ulcers. Intrinsic factors alter the structural components of, and the blood supply to, the tissues or reduce the sensation or perception response mechanism, for example, diabetic neuropathy where a patient may not feel the stimulus to change position when pressure is applied. Poor nutritional status is frequently cited as one of these intrinsic factors (Breslow, 1991; Bergstrom *et al*, 1992; Breslow and Bergstrom, 1994; Selvaag *et al*, 2002), although, the exact mechanism by which it contributes to pressure ulcer development is poorly understood.

There is a lack of research of sound methodological quality that relates to malnutrition and pressure ulcers. Nevertheless, healthcare providers commonly associate poor nutrition with the development of pressure ulcers and also with poor healing if a pressure ulcer does develop. Malnutrition is frequently found in these patients, and up to 50% have been found to be malnourished on admission to hospital (Stratton *et al*, 2003).

Pressure ulcers result in a huge strain on resources for the health service, which is arguably 95% preventable (National Pressure Ulcer Advisory Panel [NPUAP], 2001), not to mention the human cost in terms of reduced quality of life, pain and suffering (Strauss and

Margolis, 1996). The exact pathophysiology of pressure ulcer formation is not fully understood. Theories include cell deformation theory, ischaemia-reperfusion injury and cell-to-cell contact theory (Bouten *et al*, 2003). Research in animals has found that typical ischaemia-reperfusion damage can be prevented in part by treatment with vitamin E (Houwing *et al*, 2000). However, further research is necessary to determine whether these results can be extrapolated to humans.

This chapter seeks to investigate the role of nutrition in the prevention of pressure ulcers and will focus on the effect of mixed nutritional support on pressure ulcer development in at-risk groups and on nutritional status as a predictor of pressure ulcer development with specific reference to albumin. Low serum albumin is frequently cited as a nutritional risk factor for pressure ulcer development, however, other aetiologies of hypoalbuminaemia are often not considered which has resulted in confusion and controversy (Finucane, 1995; Gilmore *et al*, 1995; Anthony *et al*, 2000).

The literature accessed for this chapter was obtained using CINAHL and Medline. Key terms to facilitate the search were 'pressure ulcer', 'decubitus ulcer', 'pressure sore', 'bed sore', 'malnutrition', 'nutritional status' and 'nutrition support'. Hand searching also supplemented the evidence base. A paucity of good quality clinical trials was found and several of the studies cited are from before 2000.

Effect of nutritional status on pressure ulcer development

Allman *et al* (1995) conducted a prospective cohort study of pressure ulcer risk factors among 286 patients admitted to an acute hospital. Inclusion criteria included that they were expected to be chair- or bed-bound for at least five days, or had a hip fracture and were over 55 years of age. Of the subjects, 12.9% developed a grade 2 pressure ulcer or above. They found after multivariate Cox regression analysis that lymphopenia and decreased body weight were independent nutritional risk factors. Lymphopenia, defined as lymphocyte counts less than $1.5 \times 10^9/L$, resulted in almost five times the risk of developing a grade 2 pressure ulcer or higher. A body weight in the lowest quartile of baseline weight ($< 58\,kg$) increased pressure ulcer risk two-fold.

Haemoglobin level, food intake, hypoalbuminaemia, nurse assessment of patient build, and reduced protein or calorie intake were not found to be associated with pressure ulcer development.

Conversely, Anthony *et al* (2000) suggested that albumin levels are an accurate predictor of pressure ulcer risk and recommended that risk assessment of pressure ulcers can possibly be improved by adding serum albumin to one of the pre-existing pressure ulcer risk assessment tools such as the Waterlow score. Using logistic regression, they found hypoalbuminaemia to be predictive of pressure ulcers (P=0.009). However, only 6.3% of the 773 patients studied actually had a low serum albumin and the effect of confounding factors such as hepatic disease, renal disease, hydration status or diuretic usage on serum albumin was not taken into account (Thompson and Fuhrman, 2005).

Goode *et al* (1992) investigated the contribution of specific nutritional deficiencies (as indicated by zinc, vitamin A, C and E, albumin and haemoglobin concentrations) to the risk of developing pressure ulcers in 21 older patients with fractured neck of femur in an observational cohort study. They concluded that low concentrations of leucocyte vitamin C are a risk factor for pressure ulcer development in this patient group. Due to the very small sample size, the results of this study are not statistically significant, nevertheless, this research warrants further investigation in a much larger study.

Ek *et al* (1991) investigated the development of pressure ulcers in a cohort of 501 patients admitted to a long-term medical ward and who remained in hospital for more than three weeks. From this they found 28.5% of subjects to be malnourished. Furthermore, they found that the pressure ulcer frequency was higher among the malnourished group with 34.8% of them developing pressure ulcers compared with 20.6% in the non-malnourished group (p<0.01). Following multiple regression analysis, serum albumin (p<0.001), mobility (p<0.001), and activity and food intake (p<0.05) were found to be the most useful predictors of pressure ulcer development.

However, a description of a power calculation was not cited in the study report. Therefore, it is questionable that these results reached true statistical significance. Additionally, only about one-third of patients initially included in the study could be followed up for the full study period of 26 weeks, due to earlier discharge or death. The assessment of food intake was vague and subjective. Intake is simply described as 'normal, insufficient, parenteral or no intake'. This method gives no indication of the nutrient quality of the diet consumed. Albumin, yet again is found to be a predictor of pressure ulcers. However, was the low albumin due to malnutrition or was it due to other disease processes which were not controlled for in this study? Despite these limitations, this study supports the evidence that malnutrition, as measured by traditional assessment techniques, is a contributing factor to pressure ulcer development.

Pinchcofsky-Devin and Kaminsky (1986) concluded in their cross-sectional study of 232 nursing home patients that serum albumin and total lymphocyte count were accurate predictors of pressure ulcer development because they are accurate markers of malnutrition. This study is frequently cited as evidence that malnutrition contributes to pressure ulcer development (Bergstrom *et al*, 1992; Finucane, 1995; Lewis, 1998). They suggested that if the serum albumin is below 3.3 g/dL and the total lymphocyte count is below 1220 mm^3, nutritional intervention should be implemented to prevent pressure ulcer development. They disregarded the fact that the other biochemical measures of nutritional status, serum prealbumin and retinol binding protein were not significantly lower in the group with pressure ulcers compared with the group without, despite these parameters being measured. Also, they did not cite the anthropometric measures of either group, although several measures were taken. Therefore, they based their nutritional assessment on only two parameters, which are neither highly sensitive nor specific to malnutrition (Thompson and Fuhrman, 2005).

In addition, they extrapolated that as severe malnutrition (as they defined it) was present in all the patients who already had pressure ulcers, that it was a risk factor for their development. They did not consider that the pressure ulcer could have caused the malnutrition. Albumin levels could have been lowered due to an acute inflammatory response, infection or losses through exudate (Berlowitz and Wilking, 1989; Thomas, 2001). They discovered an inverse relationship between the grade of the ulcer and the serum albumin, deducing that as the ulcer worsened, the patient became more malnourished. Albumin may be a good marker of disease severity but this is not necessarily related to malnutrition (Thompson and Fuhrman, 2005).

Berlowitz and Wilking (1989) highlighted the pitfalls of relying too much on information gleaned from cross-sectional studies. They undertook a comparison of a cohort study with a cross-sectional study in the same population at a chronic care hospital. First, a cross-sectional analysis identified factors associated with the presence of pressure ulcers. Cohort methodology was then used to identify factors associated with the future development of a pressure ulcer.

Following multivariate analysis of the cross-sectional data (n = 299), the odds of having a pressure ulcer were almost twice as much for those with impaired nutritional intake (odds ratio [OR] = 1.9) and for every

10 mg/ml decrease in the serum albumin, the odds of having a pressure ulcer doubled.

Twenty of the 185 patients in the cohort analysis developed a pressure ulcer (11%). Once again, impaired nutritional intake was found to be a significant (p < 0.05) independent predictor for the future development of a pressure ulcer (OR = 2.8). However, hypoalbuminaemia was not associated with pressure ulcer development. This illustrates the importance of interpreting cross-sectional studies carefully. They can be subject to considerable bias. For example, albumin was not routinely measured but was more frequently measured in the patients with a pressure ulcer present on admission and on all those that developed a pressure ulcer. Several cross-sectional studies have found that patients with pressure ulcers have low serum albumin. This study supports the theory that the low serum albumin associated with pressure ulcers is a secondary factor. The pressure ulcer causes the low serum albumin, rather than vice versa.

Mixed nutritional supplementation and pressure ulcer development

A Cochrane review has found the evidence to support the use of nutritional supplementation in the treatment of pressure ulcers to be inconclusive due to the poor methodological quality of the research undertaken so far (Norris and Reynolds, 1971; Taylor and Rimmer, 1974; Chernoff et al, 1990; ter Riet et al, 1995; Langer et al, 2003). However, the review found weak evidence to support the use of mixed nutritional supplements in the prevention of pressure ulcers (Langer et al, 2003).

Hartgrink et al (1998) undertook a randomised controlled trial in 140 patients who had a fractured hip and were at high risk of developing a pressure ulcer. The experimental group received the standard hospital diet and an additional one litre of nasogastric overnight tube feeding providing 1500 kcal and 60 g protein. The control group received the hospital diet alone. Of the 62 tube-fed patients, only 25 accepted their tube for more than one week and 16 patients for two weeks. Therefore, this trial was too small to detect statistically significant differences.

The authors concluded that the nasogastric feeding was poorly tolerated and although the incidence and severity of pressure ulcers decreased in the tube-fed group, this difference was not significant. However, energy and protein intake, total serum protein, haemoglobin and serum albumin were significantly higher in the group receiving tube feeding after one and two weeks.

There were several limitations to this study: there was no blinding as a placebo was considered unethical; despite the high attrition rate, no intention to treat analysis was performed; and the method of randomisation was not described. Nonetheless, this study was useful in that it demonstrated that nasogastric feeding is not well tolerated in this patient group and other modes of nutritional support should be considered in future research.

Houwing *et al* (2003) undertook a double-blind, randomised controlled trial of 103 hip fracture patients. The intervention group received the standard hospital diet and two 200 ml oral supplements providing a total of 500 kcal, 40g protein, 6 g L-arginine, 20 mg zinc, 500 mg vitamin C, 200 mg vitamin E and 4 mg carotenoids. The control group received the standard hospital diet and two 200 ml non-calorific water-based placebo drinks. Patients were followed up for 28 days. They found that 59% of the placebo group developed a grade 1–2 pressure ulcer compared with 55% in the intervention group (p=0.420). The incidence of grade 2 pressure ulcers alone was 18% in the intervention group and 28% in the control group (p=0.345). Time of onset showed a trend (p=0.090) towards a delayed onset of pressure ulcer in the supplemented group (3.6±0.9 days) compared with the placebo group (1.6±0.9 days).

The authors concluded that nutritional supplementation of this group may delay the onset and progression of pressure ulcers. If the supplementation had been started earlier (median start day was two days after surgery and 57% of the group developed their pressure ulcer in the first two days and 76% by the fourth day after surgery), it may have been able to reduce the pressure ulcer incidence significantly. It is well documented that a significant amount of damage is done before signs show on the skin surface (Bouten *et al*, 2003).

Yet again, the study was far too small to detect any clinically important difference as statistically significant. A power calculation showed that 350 patients would be needed per group in order to detect a 25% difference in pressure ulcer incidence (Langer *et al*, 2003).

Delmi *et al* (1990) undertook a randomised controlled trial involving 59 patients with femoral neck fractures in an orthopaedic unit of a hospital in Geneva. The intervention group (n=27) received a daily 250 ml oral nutrition supplement providing 254 kcal, 20.4 g protein, 29.5 g carbohydrate and 58 g fat. It also contained an extensive range of vitamins, minerals and trace elements. They received this in addition to the standard hospital diet. The control group (n = 32) received the standard hospital diet only. Groups were followed up for up to six months.

The authors suggest that nutritional supplementation reduces pressure ulcer incidence as well as several other complications. Again, this study was not large enough to provide conclusive evidence and had several flaws in its methodology.

Despite a lack of statistical significance due to small sample sizes, all the studies detailed above reported a lower incidence of pressure ulcers in the supplemented groups.

In an additional part to Ek *et al*'s study (1991), a randomised controlled trial investigating the effect of nutritional supplementation on the development of pressure ulcers in the same patient group was undertaken. Subjects were randomised into either the intervention group (who received two 200 ml supplements each containing 8 g protein, 8 g fat, 200 kcal and 24 g carbohydrate in addition to the standard 2200 kcal per day hospital diet) or the control group (who received the hospital diet alone).

They found no statistically significant difference in pressure ulcer development between those who received nutritional support and those who did not. Perhaps no reduction in pressure ulcer development was noted in the group who received supplements because there was poor compliance with the sip feeds or because they reduced voluntary oral intake. Unfortunately, we cannot tell this from the study.

Bourdel-Marchasson *et al* (2000) conducted a multicentre, randomised controlled trial with 672 patients older than 65 years in the acute phase of a critical illness. Patients in the nutritional intervention group received two oral supplements per day in addition to the standard 1800 kcal per day hospital diet. The comparison group received the standard hospital diet alone. Each 200 ml supplement provided 200 kcal, 15 g protein, 4.4 g fat, 25 g carbohydrate, 15 mg vitamin C and 1.8 mg of zinc. Patients were followed up for 15 consecutive days or until discharge if that came first.

At 15 days, the cumulative incidence of pressure ulcers was 40% (118/295) in the nutritional intervention group versus 48% (181/377) in the control group. This equates to a relative risk of developing an ulcer while taking oral nutrition support of 0.83 (95% CI: 0.70–0.99). The authors undertook multivariate analysis to account for differences in baseline comparability and found that patients receiving the intervention were significantly less likely to develop a pressure ulcer. Low serum albumin was also found to be an independent risk factor.

This is the largest randomised controlled trial investigating the effect of nutritional support on pressure ulcer incidence that is also of satisfactory methodological quality. It provides evidence that older people recovering from illness appear to develop fewer pressure ulcers when given nutritional supplementation. Unfortunately, from this study we cannot deduce what part of the sip feed provided the benefit. Was it due simply to the extra energy or was it one of the micronutrients that protected the skin integrity?

Conclusion

Confusion exists surrounding the role of albumin as a predictor of pressure ulcer risk and as a marker of nutritional status. Serum albumin level can help to identify chronic malnutrition when used in conjunction with other nutritional parameters (Thompson and Fuhrman, 2005).

Alone, it lacks the specificity and sensitivity required to identify malnutrition accurately. It has been hypothesised that low albumin is a risk factor for pressure ulcer development, as it can cause cellular dehydration and interstitial oedema (Allman *et al*, 1995). However, from the evidence reviewed, low serum albumin appears to be a secondary factor in pressure ulcer development rather than a causative one, and may act as a good marker of wound severity and wound progress. However, we cannot assume that the low albumin is due to malnutrition. As hypoalbuminaemia has been found to be a marker of morbidity and mortality, it could indirectly identify those at highest nutritional risk (Yearick *et al*, 1980).

There is evidence that elderly people recovering from illness benefit from oral mixed nutritional supplements, but the evidence to support their use in other groups is inconclusive. That is not to say that the benefits do not exist. It may just be difficult to demonstrate due to the inherent limitations of nutrition research and it may reflect the poor methodological quality and small sample sizes of the studies undertaken to date.

The clinical trials tend to be heterogeneous with regard to patients and interventions, with different primary outcomes being evaluated making it difficult to come to a balanced conclusion. Adequately powered trials with rigorous methodology are necessary.

Pressure ulcers result from a complex interaction of factors, malnutrition being one. Malnutrition is very unlikely to be the sole cause but can compromise tissue integrity. When combined with other risk factors as well as pressure, shear and/or friction, it may lead to a pressure ulcer in a person who otherwise would not have developed one.

It is worth highlighting that however small a contributing factor malnutrition may be, unlike so many other risk factors, it is potentially reversible. As pressure ulcers tend to develop within the first few days of admission to hospital, early nutritional screening is essential to allow for early intervention. This could be included in a pressure ulcer risk assessment tool. A reliable and validated tool such as the Malnutrition Universal Screening Tool (MUST) should be used (Elia, 2003). Appropriate staff should be trained in nutritional screening and nutritional management of patients identified as at risk of malnutrition. Very high-risk patients and those with complex nutritional needs should be referred to a registered dietitian for a comprehensive nutritional assessment and an individualised dietetic treatment plan.

References

Allman R, Goods P, Patrick M (1995) Pressure ulcer risk factors among hospitalised patients with activity limitation. *JAMA* **273**: 865–70

Anthony D, Reynolds T, Russell L (2000) An investigation into the use of serum albumin in pressure sore prediction. *J Adv Nurs* **32**(2): 359–65

Bergstrom N, Braden M, Laguzza A Holman V (1992) A prospective study of pressure sore risk among institutionalised elderly. *J Am Geriatr Soc* **40**: 747–58

Berlowitz D, Wilking S (1989) Risk factors for pressure sores. A comparison of cross-sectional and cohort-derived data. *J Am Geriatr Soc* **37**(11): 1043–50

Bourdel-Marchasson I, Barateau M, Rondeau V, *et al* (2000) A multicentre trial of the effect of oral nutrition supplementation in critically ill older patients. *Nutrition* **16**(1): 1–5

Bouten C, Oomens C, Baaijens F, Bader D (2003) The etiology of pressure ulcers: skin deep or muscle bound. *Arch Phys Med Rehabil* **84**: 616–19

Breslow R (1991) Nutritional status and dietary intake of patients with pressure ulcers: a review of the literature 1943–1989. *Decubitus* **4**: 16–21

Breslow R (1993) The importance of dietary protein in healing pressure ulcers. *J Am Geriatr Soc* **41**(4): 357–62

Breslow R, Bergstrom N (1994) Nutritional prediction of pressure ulcers. *J Am Diet Assoc* **94**: 1301–4

Chernoff R, Milton K, Lipschitz D (1990) The effect of high protein formula (Replete) on decubitus ulcer healing in long-term tube-fed institutionalised patients. *J Am Diet Assoc* **90**: A–130

Delmi M, Rapin C, Bengoa J (1990) Dietary supplementation in elderly patients with femoral neck fracture. *Lancet* **335**: 1013–16

Ek A-C, Unosson M, Larsson J, Von Schenck H, Bjurilf P (1991) The development and healing of pressure sores related to the nutritional state. *Clin Nutr* **10**: 245–50

Elia M (ed) (2003) *Screening for Malnutrition: A Multidisciplinary Responsibility. Development and use of the 'Malnutrition Universal Screening Tool' ('MUST') for adults. Malnutrition Advisory Group (MAG), a Standing Committee of Bapen*. BAPEN, Redditch, Worcs

European Pressure Ulcer Advisory Panel (1998) *Pressure Ulcer Treatment Guideline*. Available online at: www.epuap.org/gltreatment.html (last accessed 7th February 2007)

European Pressure Ulcer Advisory Panel (2002) *Pressure Ulcer Prevalence Monitoring Project: Summary Report on the Prevalence of Pressure Ulcers*. Available online at: www.epuap.org/review4_2/index.html (last accessed 2nd May 2006)

Finucane TE (1995) Malnutrition, tube feeding and pressure sores: data are incomplete. *J Am Geriatr Soc* **43**: 447–51

Gilmore S, Robinson G, Posthauer M (1995) Clinical indicators associated with unintentional weight loss and pressure ulcers in elderly residents of nursing home facilities. *J Am Diet Assoc* **95**(9): 984–92

Goode HF, Burns E, Walker BE (1992) Vitamin C depletion and pressure sores in elderly patients with femoral neck fracture. *Br Med J* **305**: 925–27

Hartgrink H, Wille J, Konig P, Hermans J, Brelau PJ (1998) Pressure sores and tube feeding in patients with fracture of the hip: a randomised clinical trial. *Clin Nutr* **17**: 287–92

Houwing R, Overgoor M, Jansen G, Asbeck A, Haalboom J (2000) Pressure induced skin lesions in pigs: reperfusion injury and the effects of Vitamin E. *J Wound Care* **9**(1): 36–40

Houwing R, Rozendaal M, Weseling W, Beuleus J, Buskens E, Haalboom J (2003) Assessment of the effect of nutritional supplementation on the prevention of pressure ulcers in hip fracture patients. *Clin Nutr* **22**(4): 401–5

Langer G, Schloemer G, Kner A, Kuss O, Behrens J (2003) Nutritional interventions for preventing and treating pressure ulcers (Review). *Cochrane Database Syst Rev* **3**. Art.No:C D003216. D0110.1002/14651858.Cd003216

Lewis B (1998) Nutrient intake and the risk of pressure ulcer development in older patients. *J Wound Care* 7(1): 31–5

National Pressure Ulcer Advisory Panel (2001) Pressure ulcers in America: prevalence, incidence and implications for the future: an executive summary of the National Pressure Ulcer Advisory Panel Monograph. *Adv Skin Wound Care* 14: 208–215

Norris J, Reynolds R (1971) The effect of oral zinc sulphate treatment on decubitus ulcers. *J Am Geriatr Soc* 19: 793

Pinchcofsky-Devin G, Kaminsky M (1986) Correlation of pressure sores and nutritional status. *J Am Geriatr Soc* 34: 435–40

Selvaag E, Bohmer T, Benkestock K (2002) Reduced serum concentrations of riboflavin and ascorbic acid, and blood thiamine, pyrophosphate and pyridoxal 5 phosphate in geriatric patients with and without pressure sores. *J Nutr Health Aging* 6(1): 75–7

Strauss E, Margolis D (1996) Malnutrition in patients with pressure ulcers: morbidity, mortality and clinically practical assessments. *Adv Wound Care* 9: 37–40

Stratton R, Green C, Elia M (2003) *Disease-related Malnutrition. An Evidence-based Approach to Treatment*. CABI Publishing, UK

Taylor V, Rimmer S (1974) Ascorbic acid supplementation in the treatment of pressure sores. *Lancet* 1: 544–6

ter Riet G, Kessels A, Knipschild PG (1995) Randomised clinical trial of ascorbic acid in the treatment of pressure ulcers. *J Clin Epidemiol* 48: 1453–60

Thomas B (2001) *Manual of Dietetic Practice*. Blackwell Science, London

Thompson C, Fuhrman P (2005) Nutrients and Wound Healing: Still searching for the magic bullet. *Nutr Clin Pract* 20(3): 331–47

Yearick E, Wang M, Pisias S (1980) Nutritional status of elderly: dietary and biochemical findings. *J Gerontol* 35: 663–71

CHAPTER 6

UNDERSTANDING THE CAUSES OF CHRONIC OEDEMA

Christine Moffatt

Chronic oedema affects over 100 000 people in the UK giving it a prevalence similar to that of leg ulceration. In order to offer effective treatment, it is essential that the clinician understands the varying causes of chronic oedema, and how underlying pathology influences management choices. The impact of chronic oedema on the patient's life should not be underestimated, and findings presented here underpin the importance of a rapid diagnosis and successful management, to maximise the health-related quality of life (HRQoL) for the patient.

It is only in recent years that epidemiological studies have shown that more than 100 000 people are suffering from chronic oedema in the UK due to a wide variety of causes (Moffatt *et al*, 2003) (*Figure 6.1*), such as primary lymphoedema or cardiovascular disease. These findings suggest that the problem is as common as leg ulceration, a now well-recognised health problem.

Until recently, however, little guidance has been available for professionals treating patients with varying degrees of chronic oedema (Lymphoedema Framework, 2006a), and lymphoedema has been a relatively small specialist area of practice frequently limited to the treatment of patients with cancer-related lymphoedema.

The findings of Moffatt *et al* (2003) indicate that both lymphoedema and chronic oedema are more common than initially realised. Chronic oedema particularly presents problems in the community setting, and is often a management challenge to community nurses.

To offer effective treatment, it is important to understand why chronic oedema develops as a symptom of different disease processes and to appreciate that many of the patients seen in the community by district nurses have chronic oedema due to a variety of causes.

This chapter will describe the mechanisms of oedema formation, clinical presentations, review what is known on the impact of chronic oedema on patient's lives and briefly consider current therapies for palliation of symptoms of chronic oedema.

Definitions of chronic oedema

Oedema is the accumulation of fluid in the extravascular tissue and is a symptom of many different clinical conditions, and occurs as a result of a number of complex mechanisms involving the permeability of the capillary wall and the oncotic and hydrostatic pressure gradients that exist between the blood vessels and the tissues (European Wound Management Association [EWMA], 2003). The blood capillary wall is a semi-permeable membrane and interstitial fluid moves continually between the blood capillary and the tissues.

Tissues in this space include collagen and large proteoglycan molecules. The exchange of nutrients, wastes, fluid, electrolytes and proteins from the vascular and lymphatic systems and tissue cells occurs through this space. In this area, pressure may be low and attract fluid into the tissue, or be unusually high and force fluid into the lymphatics and capillaries. It is in the interstitial fluid space that the forces resulting in oedema come into effect. The causes of different types of oedema are depicted in *Table 6.1*.

Causes of oedema

Increased capillary permeability

When inflammation occurs due to any cause, it triggers a complex interaction with the release of chemical mediators such as histamine. As a result, the capillaries become more permeable allowing fluid to accumulate in the tissues resulting in oedema. In many cases, this type of oedema is quickly resolved once the source of the inflammation (eg. sprains) is identified and treated. However, other chronic inflammatory conditions, such as arthritis, are associated with prolonged oedema that with time may lead to progressive tissue changes.

Hormonal, cyclic oedema or idiopathic oedema may present as generalised fluid and weight gain in women and may be accompanied by constipation and oliguria. This is frequently associated with the menstrual cycle (Williams and Mortimer, 2007).

Table 6.1: Chronic oedema		
Physiology	Possible cause	Effect
Increased capillary permeability	Cellulitis, arthritis, hormonal cyclic oedema	Inflammatory oedema, 'idiopathic oedema'
Increased venous (capillary) pressure	Heart failure, venous insufficiency, dependency syndrome	Cardiac, lymphovenous, dependency oedema
Increased oncotic tissue pressure	Failure of lymph drainage	Lymphoedema
Decreased oncotic capillary pressure	Hypoalbuminaemia, nephrotic syndrome, hepatic failure	Hypoproteinaemic oedema

Adapted from: Partsch H (2003) Understanding the pathophysiological effects of compression. In: European Wound Management Association (EWMA) Position Document. *Understanding Compression Therapy.* MEP Ltd, London: 2–4

Increased capillary permeability resulting in oedema is also seen in acute infections (such as cellulitis), ischaemia, burns, exposure to toxins, vitamin deficiencies and immune reactions.

Increased venous (capillary) pressure
Lymphovenous oedema

Damage to the venous circulation, such as venous obstruction occurring as a result of deep vein thrombosis (DVT), or venous pump failure, causes reflux of venous blood and a rise in pressure in the venous circulation (ambulatory venous hypertension). The resultant increase in pressure causes enlargement of the pores within the capillary wall, enabling fluid and other macromolecules to pass into the interstitium resulting in oedema. If the increased pressure is not treated, it leads to chronic venous insufficiency which, in turn, results in oedema, lipodermatosclerotic changes and varicose eczema. The fluid in the leg is at risk of infection and complex inflammatory changes may lead to ulceration in a proportion of patients with lymphovenous oedema.

DVT and post-thrombotic syndrome are associated with damage to the deep subfascial lymphatics that are linked to the damaged deep veins in patients with lymphovenous oedema (Lymphoedema Framework, 2006b). Patients with lipodermatosclerosis also develop lymphatic damage to the superficial prefascial lymph vessels in the affected area (Williams and Mortimer, 2007). Ulcerated limbs appear to have impaired lymph drainage when assessed by lymphoscintigraphy. Other studies show that there is impaired lymphatic drainage around the site of an infected venous ulcer, and that there are dermal lymphatic abnormalities in areas of atrophie blanche (Bollinger *et al*, 1982). While lymphatic changes are clearly not the main mechanism causing oedema in venous ulceration, they do, however, play an important contributory role. Furthermore, many of these patients are immobile and sit with their limbs in a dependent position, further worsening the level of oedema.

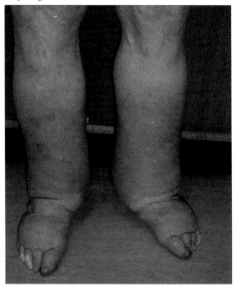

Figure 6.1: Limbs with lymphovenous oedema

Recognising the concurrent involvement of the lymphatics in venous disease is important, as it influences the way in which treatment is delivered. Compression therapy remains the cornerstone of treatment but requires an adaptation in choice of compression materials and application techniques to accommodate these changes (EWMA, 2005).

Figures 6.1 and *6.2* are two examples of patients with lymphovenous oedema. Localised swelling of the foot and toes are a frequent development in patients with venous ulcers. This type of

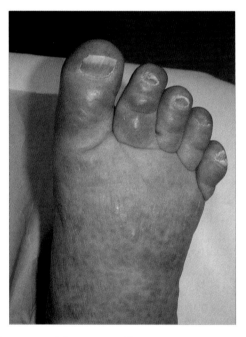

Figure 6.2: Toe swelling

swelling is probably related to the trapping of oedema in the foot and the resulting tissue changes that occur after the long-term presence of oedema. Inappropriate application of a band of high pressure around the ankle creates a tourniquet effect preventing adequate lymph drainage from the foot. Forefoot oedema develops because of trapped oedema in the toes, and tissue changes lead to fibrosis that may reduce the effectiveness of the compression that is applied. Toe swelling is a common phenomenon. Intertrigo occurs between the toes leading to bacterial entry and frequent episodes of cellulitis. These episodes lead to worsening oedema and overall deterioration of lymphatic drainage. Lymphatic involvement in the venous patient is also seen in oedema

formation in the thigh region (*Figure 6.3*). If left untreated, the tissues change from soft and pitting to fibrotic and non-pitting. Uncontrolled oedema leads to significant problems in ulcer healing (*Figure 6.4*).

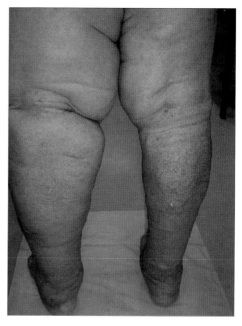

Figure 6.3: Oedema formation in the thigh region

Cardiac oedema

Increased venous pressure also occurs in patients with cardiac oedema, as the heart can no longer pump blood effectively around the body (*Figure 6.5*). Cardiac oedema may develop quickly or may be more insidious. The swelling is predominantly soft and pitting, although in patients with chronic heart failure, the tissues will eventually become fibrotic. In those who develop acute cardiac failure, the sudden increase in oedema may cause pronounced erythema and leakage of fluid from the tissues (*Figure 6.6*). Large blisters can develop that may eventually lead to ulceration. Oedema

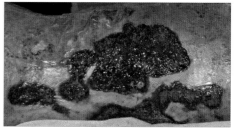

Figure 6.4: Chronic oedema associated with delayed ulcer healing

may extend to the thighs and eventually to the genitalia and sacral area. The oedema is associated with increased shortness of breath on exertion, during exercise or when lying down, and the jugular vein may be distended. Patients frequently complain of loss of appetite and feeling generally unwell and tired. Other cardiac symptoms may include atrial fibrillation. Patients frequently report a number of risk factors for cardiovascular disease, such as smoking and hypertension, and may have a history of other cardiovascular events, such as transient ischaemic attack, myocardial infarction and cerebrovascular accident.

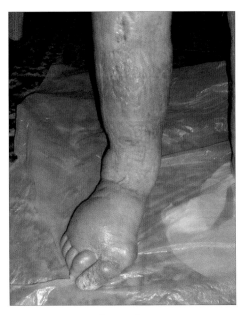

Figure 6.5: Oedema due to cardiac failure

Dependency oedema

Dependency oedema or 'armchair syndrome' occurs when the limb is kept hanging down and immobile (*Figure 6.7*). Oedema develops due to a combination of mechanisms. When the foot is dependent, pressure develops in the venous circulation (venous hypertension) leading to increased capillary permeability and oedema formation. This rise in pressure can be counteracted by periods of high elevation with the foot higher than the heart to promote drainage.

Oedema can also be reduced by activating the calf and foot

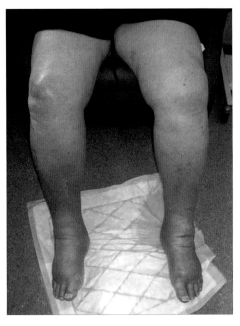

Figure 6.6: Acute cardiac oedema with erythema. Leakage of fluid can be noted on the mat below the feet

pumps. Simple flexion, dorsiflexion and circular movements of the ankle may promote this if regularly performed throughout the day. Patients who sit with their limbs in a dependent position often have other concurrent medical and mobility problems that prevent movement. Such patients frequently have complex oedema problems due to underlying chronic conditions such as cardiac and renal disease and chronic arthritis. Some of the worse cases of chronic oedema occur in those who do not go to bed at night but sit in a chair (Franks _et al_, 1995), which should be avoided at all costs.

Increased oncotic tissue pressure

Oncotic pressure has been defined as 'the osmotic pressure created by protein colloids in plasma' (Lymphoedema Framework, 2006a). Increased oncotic pressure occurs in patients with lymphoedema. Lymphoedema is defined as the accumulation of fluid and other tissue elements (subcutaneous fat, tissue protein) in the interstitial space due to insufficiency in the transport capacity of the lymphatic system (International Society of Lymphology [ISL], 2003).

Lymphoedema develops in a number of stages from mild to severe, referred to as stages 0–III (ISL, 2003):

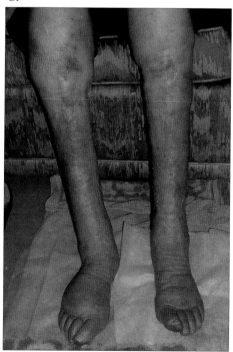

- _Stage 0:_ A sub-clinical state where swelling is not present despite impaired lymph transport. This stage may exist for months or years before any oedema becomes evident.
- _Stage I:_ This represents early onset of the condition where there is accumulation of tissue fluid that subsides with limb elevation. The oedema may be pitting.
- _Stage II:_ At this stage, limb elevation alone rarely reduces swelling and pitting is manifest.

Figure 6.7: Dependency oedema

- *Late stage II:* There may or may not be pitting as tissue fibrosis is more evident.
- *Stage III:* The tissue is hard (fibrotic) and pitting is absent. Skin changes such as thickening, hyperpigmentation, increased skin folds, fat deposits and warty overgrowths develop.

Lymphoedema manifests as swelling of one or more limbs and can include the corresponding quadrant of the trunk. Swelling can also affect the head and neck and genitalia. It is categorised as primary or secondary lymphoedema, depending on aetiology. Primary lymphoedema is the result of congenital malformation of the lymph conducting system, while secondary lymphoedema results from damage to the lymphatic vessels or lymph nodes due to trauma, disease (malignant or venous), surgery, infection, irradiation, immobility and dependency syndrome (Browse *et al*, 2003).

The oedema contains protein, water, cell debris and hyaluronan that accumulates in the interstitium. Hypertension develops in those lymphatic vessels that remain functioning. The accumulation and impaired transport of immune cells leads to chronic inflammatory changes. Chronic, recurrent episodes of cellulitis frequently occur, promoting further fibrotic tissue changes and laying down of adipose tissue. These combined effects lead to a progressive worsening of the overall condition of the patient.

Decreased oncotic capillary pressure

Decreased oncotic capillary pressure occurs in conditions where there is fluid overload/electrolyte imbalance or a decreased protein content of serum. The commonest causes are nephrotic syndrome and liver failure.

Patients who are extremely malnourished and have a very low blood albumin level may also develop severe oedema. In this situation, the imbalance between the tissue oncotic pressure (higher pressure) and the capillary oncotic pressure (lower pressure) causes fluid to be drawn into the tissues and accumulate as oedema. This type of oedema may be more generalised with ascites. Proteins such as albumin are processed in the liver and oedema occurs when the plasma protein concentration falls below 27 g/litre (Williams and Mortimer, 2007).

Outstanding questions

There are still many questions about lymphoedema and chronic oedema formation and the exact mechanisms leading to it. Researchers have prompted a review of the microcirculatory mechanisms. For example, in a study of patients with arm lymphoedema secondary to breast cancer, there was an association with increased arterial inflow and low levels of protein concentration in those who developed lymphoedema (Svensson *et al*, 1994). Other mechanisms involving angiogenic factors are also being examined in relation to this condition (Mellor *et al*, 2002).

Many of the patients being treated in the community with chronic oedema have complex clinical and psychosocial issues. The limited research that currently exists suggests that practitioners have a poor knowledge about these problems leading to incorrect or absent diagnosis and inappropriate treatment (Moffatt *et al*, 2003).

The size and complexity of the problem

The reported prevalence of lymphoedema varies due to discrepancies in its definition and measurement (Williams *et al*, 2005). With these caveats understood, the prevalence of lymphoedema following treatment for breast cancer indicates that it is a relatively common occurrence.

For example, a prevalence of 12–60% has been reported among patients with breast cancer (Mortimer *et al*, 1996; Schrenk *et al*, 2000; Ozalslan and Kuru, 2004). The figures for lymphoedema of the lower limb are less reliable and equally variable. In one retrospective study, there is a reported prevalence of 47% for lower limb lymphoedema following treatment for gynaecological cancer (Ryan *et al*, 2003a), while Hong *et al* (2002) reported a lower prevalence of 28%. Additionally, there is little published information on the prevalence of non-cancer-related lymphoedema in populations. A UK-based survey reported that 8% of 603 new referrals to 27 lymphoedema clinics over a three-month period had primary lymphoedema (Sitzia *et al*, 1998).

The lack of prevalence figures in groups other than people with cancer perpetuates the belief that this disease is the main cause of the condition. One recent study in south-west London, with a geographical population of 610000, identified at least 823 patients with lymphoedema/chronic oedema. These were patients known to health services and therefore give only a crude prevalence of 1.33/1 000 (Moffatt *et al*, 2003). This study suggests chronic oedema is a common problem in the community with at least 100 000 patients suffering with the condition in the UK.

Lymphoedema is a chronic condition. There is no cure but it is controllable with appropriate treatment and the participation of the patient in its management. If ignored, the condition can gradually deteriorate becoming increasingly more difficult to manage and taking longer to control. Lymphoedema can result in significant physical and psychological morbidity. The increase in limb size can interfere with mobility and affect body image (Tobin *et al*, 1993). In addition, pain and discomfort are physical symptoms that are frequently associated with the condition (Carroll and Rose, 1992). There are also changes in tissue structure and an increased susceptibility to frequent episodes of acute cellulitis, often resulting in frequent periods of hospitalisation and long-term dependency on antibiotics (Mortimer, 1995).

The impact of chronic oedema on patients' lives

The effects on quality of life from secondary lymphoedema associated with cancer surgery provides some insight into the problems with which patients with other causes of chronic oedema suffer. The experience of lower limb lymphoedema following surgery for gynaecological cancer is documented in a study by Ryan *et al* (2003b) in which 82 women were interviewed using a structured interview schedule. Women in this study describe being unprepared for lower limb lymphoedema and shocked by its permanence and severity. They talk of the considerable delay in finding appropriate help and having to seek out information and treatment for themselves. Many considered the information and treatment they eventually received to be inadequate and in some cases inappropriate. Referral to specialist practitioners was slow and protracted, and a large number of women implemented their own self-management strategies as a consequence. For the women in this study, lower limb lymphoedema represented a major disruption to their lives and had an impact on appearance, mobility, finances and their self-image.

In order to gain insight into the depth and complexity of the problems experienced by women with breast cancer-related lymphoedema and to explore changes in perceptions over time, Woods (1993) conducted semi-structured interviews with 37 women on referral to a specialist lymphoedema service and again six months later. At the time of referral, 90% of the women had not received even basic information about the risk of developing lymphoedema. As a consequence, the appearance of swelling brought a feeling of shock and fear that the cancer had returned, or that something had gone wrong. For some, the swelling served as a reminder of the cancer and its treatment.

Coming to terms with their lymphoedema presented particular challenges and many expressed thoughts and feelings of annoyance and frustration at the limitations imposed by the swelling. Negative body image and reduced self-confidence in their appearance were major effects forcing many to make a complete change to their preferred style of dress. The women in this study also commented that their self-confidence was negatively affected by the cumulative effects of seemingly harmless comments about their swelling by others. Woods notes that a reduction in limb volume was linked to a positive trend in the patients' perceptions of their lymphoedema. After six months of treatment some improvement was reported in coming to terms with the swelling, problems with clothes and body image and the range of movement in the swollen arm.

In a study two years later, the same author (Woods, 1995) explored the psychosocial factors that were significant for a study group of 40 women with arm swelling related to breast cancer, who were attending an established hospital-based lymphoedema clinic. Using semi-structured interviews, they found that for many women the appearance of the swelling had been unexpected and rapid, generating feelings of fear, anger and disappointment. Lack of awareness of the risk of lymphoedema and its continuing consequences was commonly expressed. Indeed, some thought it would be short-lived, that it was an effect of the cancer treatment and would go once this phase was over. Adjustment to their swollen limb and its effects was often achieved through a process of trial and error. The depth of feeling associated with such adjustment, particularly with regard to the effect of the swelling on outward appearance, was for some women considerable.

The evidence from cross-sectional and longitudinal studies using generic health-related quality of life (HRQoL) tools is that patients with lymphoedema have poorer psychological adjustment, greater deficits in their ability to function physically and socially and increased anxiety and depression than those without lymphoedema (Williams *et al*, 2004). These studies also identify that pain is a more common and dominant characteristic than is often thought to be the case. The findings indicate that pain, the frequency of acute inflammatory episodes, poor skin condition, lymphoedema in the dominant hand and reduced limb mobility are factors that can lead to deficits in HRQoL. Of equal importance is the impact that lymphoedema has on the patient. Their HRQoL is not necessarily related to the volume of the swelling, although one qualitative study has suggested it may contribute to more positive perceptions in self-image (Woods, 1993). Poor social support and maladaptive coping styles are associated with psychological and social distress, as well as with reporting significantly greater pain.

Qualitative studies in particular have explored the lived experience of lymphoedema and chronic oedema and add an important dimension to our understanding of the physical and psychosocial implications of these chronic conditions. From these studies emerge accounts of patients receiving inadequate information, of poorly-informed healthcare professionals and of insufficient specialist resources. Patients also speak of shock, disappointment, anger and fear at the first appearance of the swelling, of challenges to their self-image, of the disruption to their personal, social and vocational lives and of prolonged periods of adjustment to their lymphoedema, often achieved in the absence of adequate information and support but by trial and error. They also give accounts of the costs and difficulty associated with treatment and how managing their lymphoedema can induce considerable levels of anxiety and stress (Lymphoedema Framework, 2006a).

Advances in symptom control

Although many questions about the mechanisms leading to lymphoedema and chronic oedema formation are still unanswered, there has been some progress in treatments designed to improve the symptoms that reduce quality of life. The Lymphoedema Framework (2006) international consensus document outlines best practice as it stands to date, which it describes as holistic and multidisciplinary. The approach includes exercise and movement to improve both venous and lymphatic flow, reduction of swelling through compression therapy and/or lymphatic massage techniques, skin care to treat complications caused by lymphoedema and minimise the risk of cellulitic episodes, risk reduction of lymphoedema exacerbation factors, control of pain and management of psychosocial issues. The main areas of recent advancement in the UK have been in the availability of compression products. Inelastic or short-stretch bandages are available on drug tariff (FP10/GP/10; Heenan, 2004) and are used in multilayer lymphoedema bandaging (MLLB) (Lymphoedema Framework, 2006), which is suitable for use in patients with ABPI >0.8 and <1.2, damaged or ulcerated skin, distorted limb shape, enhanced skin folds, fibrotic tissues, lymphorrhoea and limbs too large for compression garments (Osborne, 2007).

The inclusion of a cohesive, inelastic bandage onto the drug tariff has helped simplify bandaging techniques to simple spirals, while also improving the retention on the limb (Hawkins, 2001; Charles _et al_, 2003). Arterial flow and cardiac status permitting, short-stretch systems can be used for all types of chronic oedema, whereas elastic or long-stretch bandages are best reserved for venous oedema and venous ulceration compression. _Figure 6.3_ shows how lymphatic involvement in the venous patient can form in the thigh and full-leg bandaging is necessary to correct this. A standardised method of full-leg bandaging (Osborne, 2007) is now being explained to facilitate care by a wider group of practitioners, beyond the more limited numbers of specialist lymphoedema practitioners in the UK. This type of multilayer inelastic bandaging is suitable for patients with lymphovenous and early-stage lymphoedema changes in the lower limbs.

Complex lymphoedema should always be referred to a specialist lymphoedema practitioner. Once limbs have been reshaped and reduced through courses of bandaging, compression garments can be used to maintain the gain. Until 2007, lymphoedema garments, which are stiffer than conventional British standard compression hosiery classes and, therefore, more akin to the inelastic bandages, were unavailable on the drug tariff. The lymphoedema compression garments are also in the stronger compression ranges of the European compression classes.

Intermittent pneumatic compression (IPC) can be used as an adjunct to MLLB. IPC has been thought to assist by decreasing capillary filtration, thereby decreasing lymph formation, rather than by accelerating lymph return (Lymphoedema Framework, 2006). A recent advance has been made with the redesign of the conventional IPC device (Flowtron Hydroven[TM], Huntleigh Healthcare), which works proximally to distally, rather than vice versa as in conventional

IPC devices. This new pattern of intermittent compression mimics lymphatic drainage principles and may improve movement along decongested lymph vessels.

Conclusion

Chronic oedema and its consequences have been a hidden problem for many years. As we understand more about the physiological mechanisms that lead to its development, so interventions can be developed for the different patient groups that suffer with this disabling symptom. We already appreciate that chronic oedema and lymphoedema are associated with a significant reduction in the HRQoL of patients. Improved treatment delivered within effective services is the central strategy that will help to alleviate this suffering. Professionals must continue to strive to gain the knowledge and skills to provide effective care and to ensure that chronic oedema and lymphoedema are placed firmly on the healthcare agenda, however great a challenge this appears to be.

References

Bollinger A, Paster G, Hoffmann U, Franzeck UK (1982) Fluorescence microlymphology in chronic venous incompetence. *Int Angiol* 8: 234–6

Browse N, Burnand K, Mortimer P (2003) *Diseases of the Lymphatics.* Arnold, London

Carroll D, Rose K (1992) Treatment leads to significant improvement: effect of conservative treatment on pain in lymphoedema. *Prof Nurse* 8: 32–6

Charles H, Moore C, Varrow S (2003) Cohesive short-stretch bandages in the treatment of venous leg ulceration. *Br J Community Nurs* 8(3) Suppl: 17–22

European Wound Management Association (2005) (EWMA) Focus Document. *Lymphoedema Bandaging in Practice.* MEP, London

European Wound Management Association (2003) (EWMA) Position Document. *Understanding Compression Therapy.* MEP, London

Franks PJ, Moffatt CJ, Connolly M, *et al* (1995) Factors associated with healing leg ulceration with high compression. *Age Ageing* 24: 407–10

Hawkins J (2001) A new cohesive bandage and its application. *Br J Nurs* 10(4): 249–53

Heenan A (2007) *Bandages on the Drug Tariff.* Available online at: <u>www.</u>

worldwidewounds.com/2004/march/Heenan/Tariff-Bandages.html (last accessed 24 October 2007)

Hong JH, Tsai CS, Lai CH, *et al* (2002) Postoperative loe pelvic radiation for stage I-IIA cervical cancer patients with risk factors other than pelvic lymph node metastasis. *Int J Radiat Biol Phys* 53: 1284–90

International Society of Lymphology (2003) The diagnosis and treatment of peripheral lymphedema. Consensus document of the International Society of Lymphology. *Lymphology* 36(2): 84–91

Lymphoedema Framework (2006a) *Best Practice for the Management of Lymphoedema. International Consensus*. MEP Ltd, London

Lymphoedema Framework (2006b) *Template for Practice: compression hosiery in lymphoedema*. MEP Ltd, London

Mellor RH, Stanton AWB, Menadue L, *et al* (2002) Evidence for dermal angiogenesis in breast cancer related lymphoedema demonstrated using dual site fluorescence angiography. *Microcirculation* 9: 207–19

Moffatt CJ, Franks PJ, Doherty DC, *et al* (2003) Lymphoedema: an underestimated health problem. *Q J Med* 96(10): 731–8

Mortimer PS, Bates DO, Brassington HD, *et al* (1996) The prevalence of arm oedema following treatment for breast cancer. *Q J Med* 89: 377–80

Mortimer PS (1995) Managing lymphoedema. *Clin Exp Dermatol* 20: 98–106

Osborne K (2007) Principles of below- and above-knee inelastic multilayer bandaging. *Wounds UK (Supplement)* 3(2): S29–S34

Ozalslan C, Kuru B (2004) Lymphoedema after treatment of breast cancer. *Am J Surg* 187: 69–72

Ryan M, Stainton MC, Slaytor EK, Jaconelli C, Watts S, Mackenzie P (2003a) Aetiology and prevalence of lower limb lymphoedema following treatment for gynaecological cancer. *Aust N Z J Obstet Gynaecol* 42(2): 148–51

Ryan M, Stainton MC, Jaconelli C, Watts S, Mackenzie P, Mansberg T (2003b) The experience of lower limb lymphoedema for women after treatment for gynaecologic cancer. *Oncol Nurs Forum* 30(3): 417–23

Schrenk P, Reiger R, Shamiyeh A, Wayand W (2000) Morbidity following sentinel lymph node biopsy versus axillary lymph node dissection from patients with breast carcinoma. *Cancer* 88: 608–14

Sitzia J, Woods M, Hine P, Williams A, Eaton K, Green G (1998) Characteristics of new referrals to twenty-seven lymphoedema treatment units. *Eur J Cancer* 7: 255–62

Svensson WE, Mortimer PS, Tohno E, Cosgrove DO (1994) Increased arterial flow demonstrated by Doppler ultrasound in arm swelling following breast cancer treatment. *Eur J Cancer* 30: 661–4

Tobin MB, Lacey HJ, Meyer L, Mortimer PS (1993) The psychological morbidity of breast cancer related arm swelling. *Cancer* 72: 3248–52

Williams AF, Mortimer P (2007) Lymphoedema of the lower limb: causation, assessment and management. In: Morison MJ, Moffatt CJ, Franks PJ, eds. *Leg Ulcers. A Problem-based Learning Approach.* Mosby, Elsevier, Edinburgh

Williams AF, Franks PJ, Moffatt CJ (2005) Lymphoedema: estimating the size of the problem. *Palliative Med* 19: 300–13

Williams AF, Moffatt CJ, Franks PJ (2004) A phenomenological study of the lived experience of people with lymphoedema. *Int J Palliative Nurs* 10(6): 279–86

Woods M (1993) Patient's perceptions of breast-cancer-related lymphoedema. *Eur J Cancer Care* 2: 125–8

Woods M (1995) Sociological factors and psychosocial implications of lymphoedema. *Int J Palliative Care* 1(1): 17–20

Chapter 7

Stoma-related skin complications

Angela Vujnovich

There are no definitive figures for the number of people living in the United Kingdom (UK) with a stoma. Lee (2001) suggests there are approximately 100 000 people in the UK with a stoma. The Boston Consulting Group (2005) using data based from IMS Health Incorporated Group estimates approximately 102 000 people are living in the UK with a permanent stoma. This figure is based on permanent stomas without estimating the number of temporary stomas at any one time. The actual number of people living in the UK with a stoma may be far higher then previously thought.

Each year new stomas are formed. The Department of Health (2005) estimated between 70 000–100 000 people in the UK had colorectal or urological surgery that resulted in the stoma. However, in a 12-month period from June 2006 to July 2007, IMS Health Incorporated Group (2007) recorded that there were approximately 22 000 new stomas formed in Great Britain. This is based on figures sent in from participating hospitals. This figure was made up of 11 500 new colostomies, 9200 new ileostomies and 1700 new urostomies (IMS Health Incorporated Group, 2007). Previously, most stomas were permanent. As newer surgical techniques that save anal sphincters have developed and evolved, it is now estimated that it is an even 50% split between permanent and temporary stomas. IMS Health Incorporated Health Group (2007) figures for June 2006 to July 2007 show 48% of new stomas in Great Britain were temporary. The average length of time that a patient will have a temporary stoma for is approximately nine months (IMS Health Incorporated Group, 2007).

Patients may undergo stoma-forming surgery for a variety of reasons, including:

- cancer of the bowel or bladder
- inflammatory bowel disease
- diverticular disease
- familial adenomatous polyposis
- ischaemic bowel
- obstruction
- incontinence
- abdominal or rectal trauma
- congenital malformations.

As with any surgery, there is always a risk of complications. With stoma-forming surgery, there is not only an immediate surgical risk such as post-operative haemorrhage or infection, but also the risk of a stoma-related complication. Stoma-related complications can develop immediately after surgery or can develop several months or years later. It has been reported that 47% of stoma patients will suffer at least one stoma complication (Lyon and Smith, 2001). Shellito (1998) suggested that the greatest risk of developing a stoma-related complication is usually within the first five years following surgery. Arumugan *et al* (2003) reported that 50% of patients had developed one or more complications within twelve months after stoma-forming surgery. Therefore, any patient who has a stoma formed, whether it is temporary or permanent, is at risk of developing a stoma-related complication.

Stoma-related complications include:

- parastomal hernia
- stoma retraction
- stenosis of the stoma
- prolapse of the stoma
- parastomal granulomas
- mucocutaneous separation.

While these complications are fairly common, by far the most common stoma-related complication is a skin-related one.

A review of the literature will find figures ranging anywhere from 5% (Shellito, 1998) to 42% (Borwell, 1996); with Lyon *et al* (2000) suggesting that 73% of people with a stoma will self-report a skin-related complication.

While a minor skin problem may not at first appear to have any serious consequences, it is important to remember that intact skin is essential for the normal use of a stoma appliance (Smith *et al*, 2002). Any area of skin that has become excoriated, is weeping or bleeding, can cause the stoma appliance to leak. This, in turn, causes the skin to deteriorate further, causing appliance leaks, hence, the vicious cycle continues. The patient will lose confidence in the appliance they are using if it leaks frequently, which will have a major impact on their activities of daily living and physiological well-being. Patients may report being too scared to leave their house for fear of the appliance leaking.

Skin excoriation can occur at any time and for many reasons (McKenzie and Ingram, 2001). Dermatitis from stoma effluent repeatedly leaking onto the skin is the single most common cause of peristomal skin complications (Lyon and Beck, 2001). Patients who present with a skin complication will usually be suffering from one of the following:

- faecal/urine dermatitis
- trauma
- infection
- pre-existing skin conditions.

Within each of these categories there will be different causes. Each will have different signs and symptoms that will affect individual patients in various ways, as well as having different modes of treatment.

Education of the patient with a new stoma in the immediate post-operative phase can minimise the risk of potential skin problems arising (Vujnovich, 2004). A trained stoma care nurse (SCN) based in the hospital usually undertakes this. However, as most skin complications will develop after the patient has been discharged from hospital, district and practice nurses will encounter people with a stoma in the community who are experiencing problems.

This chapter will focus on faecal or urinary skin excoriation, as this is the most common cause of stoma-related skin complaints. Trauma and allergy will also be mentioned. Treatment for faecal or urinary skin complaints can be commenced by a healthcare professional in the community with some knowledge of stoma and skin care. In instances where treatment has been commenced with no signs of improvement, the patient should be referred to their stoma care nurse. Skin complaints such as infections and pre-existing skin conditions should be referred to a stoma care nurse or dermatologist, as often the treatment required can impair the adherence of stoma appliances, leading to secondary skin complications.

Faecal or urine dermatitis

Faecal irritant reactions are more common around ileostomies than colostomies, due to the corrosive nature of the effluent. In one study on patients with permanent stomas, peristomal skin disorders were found in 57% of patients with an ileostomy, 48% of patients with a urostomy and 35% of patients with a colostomy (Herlufsen *et al*, 2006). Of those diagnosed with a skin disorder, 77% could be related to contact with stoma effluent (Herlufsen *et al*, 2006).

The effluent of ileostomies is strongly alkaline and contains unabsorbed waste products and enzymes that break down protein. Protein is a major constituent of the outermost layers of the skin and protects the skin from harmful substances. The stratum corneum is resistant to quite acidic fluid, but it is more vulnerable to alkaline substances (Stevens and James, 2003). The digestive enzymes in the alkaline effluent of an ileostomy can dissolve the protein keratin, which is found in the skin (Vujnovich 2004).

Urine that is in prolonged contact with the skin will lead to maceration in patients with a urostomy (Collett, 2002). Ideally, urinary pH should be slightly acidic and range between 6–7.5 (Fillingham and Douglas, 1997). An alkaline urinary pH of 7–8 can lead to complications with the peristomal skin and stoma, such as stomal bleeding, ulceration, urinary tract infections, odour and urinary calculi (Fillingham and Douglas, 1997). Eventually, stoma stenosis, pseudoepithelial hyperplasia and hyperkeratosis may occur (Walsh, 1992).

Patient and skin assessment

When first encountering a patient who says that they have excoriated skin, it is important to take a thorough history of the problem. Asking appropriate questions will often give numerous clues as to the cause of their skin complaint (Vujnovich, 2004) (*Table 7.1*).

All questions should be fully explored to gain a better understanding of the skin complication. Once you have completed taking a history, the next step should be a physical examination of the patient.

Start by looking at the patient's abdomen with the appliance still on. Observe the patient in different positions. Watch how the appliance changes, moves and moulds to the contours of the patient's shape in these different positions. Some appliances may be too rigid

Table 7.1: History of skin problems

Questions to ask	Rationale
When did this problem first appear?	Indicates how long the problem has been present
Has the appearance of the excoriation changed?	The excoriation may be improving or worsening, changes may indicate different stages of excoriation
Have you had this problem or any problem with your skin before?	May suggest past history of pre-existing skin problems
What treatment did you try last time or this time?	Previous treatment that may have been effective in the past, may be effective this time
Do you notice leakage at particular times?	Problems may only be reported at particular times (ie. during exercise, at night, when sitting)
What appliance are you using?	Is this appliance appropriate now?
Are you using any accessories with your stoma appliance?	Allergies are common to accessories rather than stoma appliances
How many times a day/week do you change your appliance?	May indicate too frequent appliance changes or leaving the appliance in place for too long
How many leaks a week do you experience?	Vicious circle of frequent leaks causing deterioration in skin, causing further leaks
How many times a day do you empty your appliance?	Stoma output may be high, the appliance may get too full before emptying, causing drag on the skin
Has the stoma effluent changed?	Stoma output may have increased, become looser

for the shape of the patient's abdomen. Skin folds may develop on moving, causing the appliance to lift slightly off the skin, allowing stoma effluent to seep underneath.

It is then important to watch the patient change their stoma appliance. Pay particular attention to how the patient removes the appliance and how they clean and dry their skin. If the patient is roughly pulling their appliance off, this may cause trauma to the skin; likewise, over-vigorous cleaning can damage the skin by removing the outer protective layers.

Once the appliance is off, look carefully at the back of the base plate to assess where any leakage or seepage of effluent has been occurring, subsequently affecting this area of skin. Visible tracks of effluent on the base plate will indicate where stoma effluent has been on the skin.

Now, carefully examine the area surrounding the stoma. The

distribution of the excoriation will be determined by the leakage of the stoma effluent on the skin. For the skin to become excoriated it must be in contact with faeces or urine. Pull apart any skin folds to see if the excoriation is present in the folds. View the patient's abdomen with the appliance off in different positions, such as sitting and standing, looking for skin creases that develop.

Diagnosing the cause

Your history-taking and physical assessment should have given you clues as to the underlying cause of the skin excoriation. Faecal or urine excoriation will be caused by:

- remodelling of stoma
- poorly-sited stoma
- poorly-shaped stoma
- retracted stoma.

Remodelling of stoma

Most newly-formed stomas are oedematous immediately after surgery. Over the first six to eight weeks this oedema will reduce and the stoma will remodel itself. It is important that a new stoma is measured at least weekly in the first two months. This ensures that the appliance aperture is cut to the correct size for the stoma. It is ideal to see 2–3 mm of skin around the stoma. This provides the skin with maximum protection from the corrosive fluid, but is not too tight for the stoma to be damaged by a tight-fitting appliance.

Signs of peristomal skin excoriation:

- ❖ Well-defined erythema.
- ❖ Oedema may be present.
- ❖ Blister formation.
- ❖ Areas of denuded skin.
- ❖ In severe cases there may be necrosis.
- ❖ The patient may describe a burning sensation at the site.
- ❖ Itching.

Usually after eight weeks the stoma has stopped remodelling and pre-cut appliances can be ordered.

During your physical examination you may notice an area of excoriated skin directly round the stoma. The area may appear red and angry, areas of skin may be missing and shallow superficial ulcers and dried blood may be present. Patients will complain of pain or a burning sensation at the site. This may be at the circumference of the stoma or to one side. A circumferential ring of excoriated skin would indicate that the patient is cutting the aperture in the appliance too large for the stoma, allowing skin to be exposed to faecal or urinary effluent. If the excoriation is only present in one area around the stoma, usually a crescent shape at the bottom of the stoma, it may be that the patient is not lining up the aperture with the stoma in the middle, but rather slightly off-centre, thereby exposing skin only in one place.

Poorly-sited stoma (*Figure 7.1*)

All patients having elective surgery that may result in a stoma should be seen pre-operatively by the SCN for pre-operative education, and to mark the most appropriate site of the stoma. Ideally, the patient's belt line should be avoided, the stoma should be located within the abdominal rectus muscle, all creases, skin folds, previous scars should be avoided, and the patient should be able to see the stoma when in various positions, such as sitting and standing. However, in emergency

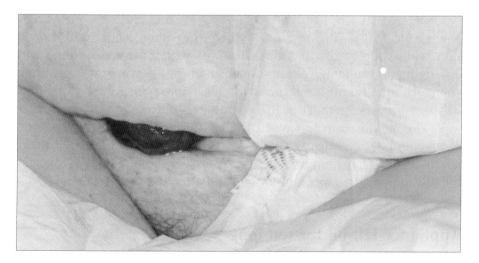

Figure 7.1: Poorly-sited stoma in skin folds

situations, pre-operative siting is not always possible and the surgeon is often faced with the dilemma of where to place the stoma. An abdomen may look flat with no skin creases when the patient is on the operating table, but will change dramatically when sitting or standing.

Poorly-shaped stoma

It is ideal for all stomas to have a spout. This is more imperative when dealing with ileostomies and urostomies than colostomies, due to the corrosive nature of the effluent. Spouts encourage the effluent to fall out and into the appliance, rather than trying to track underneath the base plate onto the skin. The optimal shape of an end ileostomy should have a spout long enough to avoid skin excoriation and should point forwards and slightly downwards (Hall *et al*, 1995). There is emerging evidence that supports a spout of an ileostomy or urostomy should be no less then 1 cm in height. In the case of a loop ileostomy, the proximal end where the effluent exits should be everted longer than the distal end (Blackley, 1998). Typically, colostomies have been constructed flush with the level of the skin. However, Nicholls (1996) advocates a spout of a few millimetres. Again, emerging evidence would suggest a colostomy height of less then 0.5 cm can lead to leakages and skin excoriation.

Retracted stoma

A retracted stoma (*Figure 7.2*) is where the stoma has shrunk into a skin fold or dip in the abdomen. Patients with a retracted stoma will usually report frequent leaks, as the output is not flowing into the stoma appliance but leaking underneath the base plate onto their skin. This will cause the skin quickly to become excoriated, leading to further leaks. Retraction can be caused by: technical difficulties at the time of operation in mobilising the bowel to reach the abdominal surface; failure to site the patient pre-operatively so that the surgeon has to guess the most appropriate position of the stoma; or, by weight gain.

Appliance left on for too long

There may be various reasons why a patient leaves their appliance on for too long. Some patients try to use fewer bags to reduce the need for further prescriptions and charges, while others may think that it only needs to be changed when it begins to leak. It should be explained to patients that prescription charges do not apply if they are over 60 years of age, in full-time education if aged 16, 17 or 18, if the stoma is permanent, or they or their partner receive income support. Patients who do not fall into these categories will be required to pay for their stoma appliances. Prescription pre-payment can help people who require large quantities or regular prescriptions, such as stoma appliances, and will save them money. Of more concern are the people who find their stoma so abhorrent that they try to ignore it, rather than face changing the appliance. These issues must be explored. Patients that are finding it difficult to come to terms with their stoma will need support and reassurance. Counselling from a trained professional may be required.

High output stoma

The normal output for an ileostomy can range from anywhere between 500–1000 mls in twenty-four hours. Anything over 1000mls is considered to be a high output. The corrosive nature of ileostomy effluent will damage the skin and erode the stoma appliance quicker. Patients may have to change their appliance more frequently, as it will start to erode if left on for long periods.

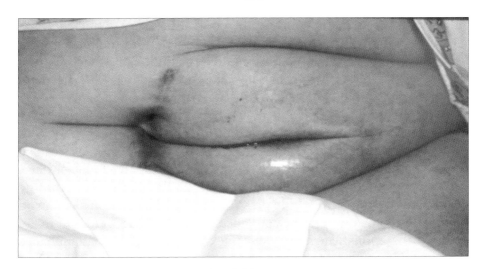

Figure 7.2: Retracted stoma in skin folds

Treatment of excoriated skin

All excoriated skin should be treated in the same way (*Figures 7.3, 7.4*). Patients should be advised to cleanse the area with warm tap water and dry thoroughly. All stomas should be re-measured using a measuring guide (usually found in the appliance box) to ensure that the aperture of the appliance is cut to the correct size. If the stoma is not round, a template of the stoma shape must be made so that the patient has the correct shape to cut the aperture to at each appliance change. It may be beneficial to use a protective barrier such as Cavilon™ No Sting Barrier Film (3M Healthcare) (Schuren *et al*, 2005). On application to the skin, Cavilon™ Film will form a waterproof barrier that will act as a protective membrane between the skin and faecal and urinary effluent. Most product companies have their own version of accessory products that can be used to treat excoriation. These are usually in the form of barrier films, which are available in sprays, creams or wipes. The other option is to use a powder. Powders are used on wet, denuded skin to dry the area and increase the adhesion of the product to the patient's skin. Care should be taken when using creams, as they can leave an oily residue on the skin and impair the adhesion of the appliance. Only a small amount, the size of a matchstick head is required. This should be thoroughly rubbed into the skin and any excess should be removed before applying the appliance. The patient should be advised to change the appliance every two days until the excoriation clears up. If the diagnosis is that the patient has been incorrectly measuring the stoma, then this treatment will heal the skin in a matter of days. However, if the stoma is poorly-sited, poorly-shaped or retracted, these measures alone will not stop the excoriation deteriorating or help it to heal, as the stoma effluent is tracking underneath the appliance causing the leakage, which then excoriates the skin (*Figure 7.5*). In these instances, the patient will need assessment from a trained SCN.

With modern developments of stoma products, situations like these can be managed conservatively without the need for further surgery to re-site or refashion the stoma. Accessories such as paste and seals can be used to build up creases to enable the appliance to stick to a flat surface. Convex appliances raise the profile of the stoma, or the end pointing downwards, by applying a little pressure around the peristomal skin and forcing the stoma out into the appliance. This encourages effluent to fall out into the appliance rather than tracking underneath the appliance onto the skin. A belt can be attached to the appliance to apply further gentle pressure to raise the profile of the stoma and hold the appliance in place. In extreme cases, paste, seals, a convex appliance and a belt may all be needed to manage conservatively the situation and prevent skin excoriation. However, in some cases, conservative management will not be successful and the stoma will require surgical refashioning or re-siting, although this does not guarantee a trouble-free stoma.

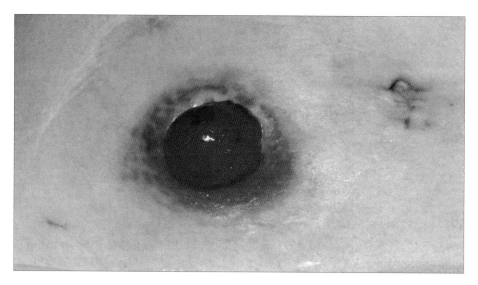

Figure 7.3: Excoriated skin, the circumference of the stoma

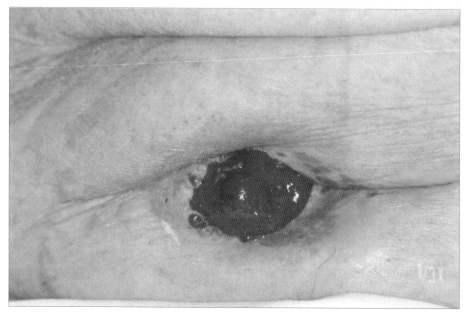

Figure 7.4: Stoma with excoriation tracking along skin crease

If the underlying cause of the excoriation is weight gain on the part of the patient, and their stoma is now retracted, it may be helpful to advise the patient to lose weight. If the stoma has sunk because of the skin folds, it may be necessary to use a convex appliance.

All patients with a high output stoma should be given a barrier protection agent, such as Cavilon™ No Sting Barrier Film, as a prophylactic agent to prevent skin excoriation, rather than treating it after it has occurred.

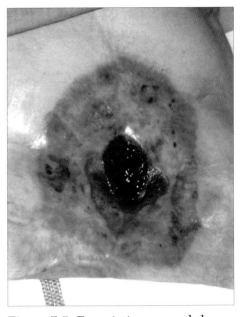

Figure 7.5: Excoriation around the stoma. Note the ulcers directly under the stoma, and to the left and right, caused by over-frequent appliance removal and over-vigorous cleaning to the area. The stoma is also flush with the skin — potentially causing effluent leakage onto the skin

Physical irritation

Physical irritation specifically refers to:

- frequent appliance changes
- poor change technique
- trauma
- radiotherapy and chemotherapy.

Frequent appliance changes

When an appliance is changed too frequently the outer skin cells that provide the skin with protection are constantly being stripped off. The skin will have a similar appearance to excoriation caused by effluence leaking onto it. It may be weeping or bleeding. Areas of skin may be denuded or ulcerated. Several companies have developed accessory products that can be used to assist patients in removing the appliance. These products can be sprayed onto the appliance, or wiped between the skin and the appliance as it is being removed. The accessory easily loosens the tackiness of the appliance making it easier to remove, thus helping to prevent repeated stripping of the outer layers of the skin.

Poor change technique

Patients should always be observed changing their appliance to assess their technique (Myers, 1996). Patients may strip their appliance off their abdomen as quickly as possible without supporting the skin. Vigorous rubbing of the skin when cleaning to ensure that all traces of effluent are removed, can also lead to damage. Some patients may have difficulty in lining up the aperture with the stoma and may be placing it off-centre, exposing the skin to effluent on one side.

Trauma

Trauma to the stoma or surrounding skin can be caused by over-vigorous cleaning and drying of the area. Rigid convexity appliances can also cause damage to the skin due to the extra pressure they create round the stoma. Patients who use a belt attachment for extra security should be advised not to wear the belt so tight that it damages the skin near the stoma causing ulcers.

Treatment of trauma

There are many different recommendations as to the frequency of appliance changes. Drainable, one-piece appliances or the base plates of two-piece appliances can be changed anywhere from every day to every four days. The average wear time is two to four days (Allen, 1998). If the peristomal skin is in excellent condition, the patient can decide what is the best routine for them. As long as their skin stays in perfect condition, this is acceptable. However, if they leave their appliance on for several days and their skin begins to deteriorate, they must change their appliance more frequently. For patients with a colostomy, it is suggested that they should change their one-piece closed appliance as necessary (Black, 2000), which may be once or twice-daily depending on their output.

A careful assessment must be taken to understand why the appliance is frequently being changed. It may simply be that the appliance is inappropriate for the stoma effluent, and changing to a more appropriate one would solve this problem. On questioning, some patients will report feeling dirty with faeces sitting in the appliance on their abdomen and they only feel clean when they change the appliance. In these cases, patients require support and advice. Explain to the patient the damage that frequent appliance changes or over-vigorous removal or cleaning and drying does to their skin, by repeatedly removing its protective layers. The use of a two-piece appliance where the patient can leave the flange in place for several days but change the bag regularly may help them to feel cleaner. Patients should be encouraged to gently remove their appliance using one hand, while the other supports the skin. The use of adhesive removers should be considered to assist in removing the appliance. The patient should demonstrate placing the new appliance in place. Two-piece appliances, where the base plate can be left in place for several days and the patient can change the bag as needed, will allow the skin to repair itself in-between base plate changes. Patients who experience difficulty lining the aperture with the stoma may find a mirror useful, or a two-piece appliance where they can line the aperture and the stoma up and then clip the bag in place. The use of rigid convexity appliances should be reviewed. There are now softer convex appliances available that still raise the profile of the stoma but cause less pressure to the surrounding peristomal skin.

Radiotherapy and chemotherapy

Skin problems related to radiotherapy and chemotherapy are relatively uncommon. Often the most common side-effect after chemotherapy and radiotherapy is diarrhoea, which can lead to appliance leakage problems and excoriated skin. When patients are experiencing diarrhoea during the course of their treatment, drainable appliances or a two-piece system (where the base plate can be left in place for several days but the bag changed as needed) should be used while the diarrhoea persists.

The severity of skin reactions after radiotherapy will depend on the total dose of radiation, the size of the area being treated, and the condition of the skin before commencing radiotherapy. Skin breakdown is most likely to occur in moist areas, skin folds, such as the groin, or in areas of recent surgery, such as the perineal region after an abdominal perineal resection (McGrath and Fulham, 2004).

Skin damage following radiotherapy can be classified as:

- *Erythema:* skin becomes pink, dry and itchy, may have a rash-like appearance or spots, and feel hot and appears similar to sunburn. Occurs two to three weeks after starting radiotherapy and resolves two to three weeks after stopping.

- *Dry desquamation:* characterised by dry, flaky, superficial skin loss which can be itchy. It is often the precursor of moist desquamation, especially if onset is early in treatment. It occurs two to three weeks after commencing therapy.
- *Moist desquamation:* skin blisters and sloughs off exposing the dermis. Raw skin may be apparent and bleeding may occur. Exudate may be serous, white, yellow or green.
- *Necrosis:* this rarely occurs (Faithful, 2001).

Patients can develop stomatitis when receiving some chemotherapy agents. These include 5-flurouracil, methotrexate, doxorubicin, bleomycin and mitomycin C. The stoma can become oedematous and inflamed. This will not cause the patient any pain, as the stoma has no nerves. Patients should be advised that they might need to adjust the aperture of their appliance to fit the oedematous stoma correctly (Porrett and McGrath, 2005).

Prevention and treatment

Any patients undergoing radiotherapy should seek advice about skin care from the centre providing their treatment. Different centres will have varying recommendations for prevention of damage. Patients should be advised to wash the skin within the treatment area with a mild soap. Moisturising creams should be applied, although alcohol, petroleum, lanolin (Korinko and Yurick, 1997), and metallic-based creams such as zinc (Lyon and Smith, 2001) should be avoided. Moisturising cream will hydrate the skin. However, care should be taken as creams can leave an oily residue impairing the adhesive of the appliance. To help soothe the erythema the moisturiser may be placed in the fridge before use. Creams should not be applied within two hours prior to treatment. If patients need to shave their abdomen so the stoma appliance adheres to the skin, they should be advised to use an electric razor rather than a wet razor while receiving radiotherapy. Perfumed products should not be used in the treatment area. Loose clothing, preferably made from natural fibres, should be worn to prevent friction over the area. Any exudate should be blotted dry with sterile gauze. Moist desquamation should not be routinely cleaned unless there is evidence of infection. Trauma of repeated cleaning will increase desquamation and damage granulating tissue.

Allergy

It is important to mention allergy, as most patients will report that their excoriated skin is due to an allergy to their appliance. An allergy can develop at any stage, even after the patient has been using the same appliance for several years with no problems (*Figure 7.6*). A true allergy to a stoma appliance is rare and only accounts for 0.6% of stoma-related skin problems (Lyon and Beck, 2001). Suspected skin allergy from stoma products can be broken down into two categories, namely, an allergy to:

- the appliance
- accessory products.

Assessment

Signs and symptoms of skin allergy include:

- erythema
- margins are indistinct and blurred and may spread beyond the area of the appliance
- blister formation
- presence of papules and vesicles
- lesions may become painfully eroded and crusted
- itching.

When examining the skin it is important to look at the distribution of the excoriation on the skin surrounding the stoma. This will often give the best clue as to the cause of the dermatitis. The skin must be in contact with the appliance to develop an allergic reaction to a stoma appliance. If the patient has skin creases, it is important to pull them apart to look for excoriation. If there is excoriation in the creases, it is likely that faeces or urine are tracking along them causing the excoriation. If the skin crease shows no signs of excoriation, an allergy may be the cause of the excoriation. While patients can develop an allergy to stoma appliances, it is more common to develop an allergy to a stoma accessory, such as a fragranced stoma bag deodoriser. In several European studies, fragrances have been demonstrated to be second only to nickel as a cause of allergic contact dermatitis (Lyon and Beck, 2001). As before, it is essential to watch the patient do a complete appliance change. The patient may be using potentially irritant substances, such as a deodoriser, perfumed cleansers, or medicated wipes.

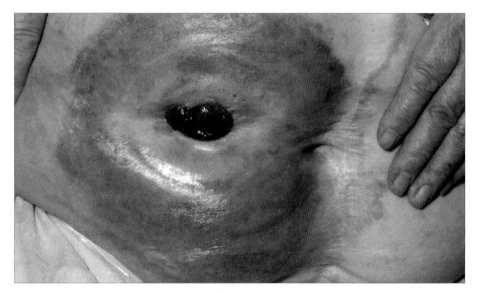

Figure 7.6: Allergy to a stoma appliance

Treatment

Patients should be advised to wash their skin with lukewarm tap water. Perfumed products should be avoided and the use of barrier preparations should only be used if advised by a clinician who has experience in the field of stoma and skin care. Any accessories the patient is using should be stopped immediately.

If an allergy to an appliance is diagnosed, the patient should change the type of appliance to one with a different adhesive, flange or wafer. True allergic dermatitis will resolve when the patient is no longer exposed to the allergen (Lyon and Beck, 2001). The application of a topical steroid to the allergy may hasten its resolution.

Testing for allergy

If an allergy is suspected, a usage test can be tried. This involves the patient placing the same appliance and any accessories they may be using on the opposite side of their abdomen to their stoma. These will be left on for several days to see if any rash develops. This test will only demonstrate that the patient is sensitive to some component of their stoma products. As allergies can develop at any stage, usage testing may be of little benefit and further investigations may be required.

Patients requiring patch or prick testing should be referred to a specialist dermatology department with experience in performing this test (Lyon and Beck, 2001). An allergy to a stoma appliance or accessory can be confirmed with a positive patch test. Appliance manufacturers are often willing to give information about compounds used in their products so that the source of the allergy can be identified and avoided in future product usage (Lawson, 2003).

Conclusions

Skin problems are common among patients with a stoma. Patients may develop a skin problem for a variety of reasons, many of which are beyond their control. Careful and thorough history-taking will often give clues as to the cause of the problem. Combine this with a careful, physical examination and a correct diagnosis can usually be swiftly made. Simple measures to treat skin excoriation can be started by healthcare professionals with a basic knowledge of stoma and skin care. In some cases, patients may need to be referred to a trained SCN for specialist advice and treatment regarding their stoma management.

References

Allen S (1998) Ileostomy. *Prof Nurse* **14**(2): 107–12

Arumugan PJ, Bevan L, MacDonald L, Watkins AJ, Morgan AR, Beynon J, Carr ND (2003) A prospective audit of stomas, analysis of risk factors and complications and their management. *Colorectal Dis* **5**(1): 49–52

Black P (2000) *Holistic Stoma Care*. Baillière Tindall, China

Blackley P (1998) *Practical Stoma Wound and Continence Management*. Research Publications Pty Ltd, Australia

Borwell B (1996) *Managing Stoma Problems*. Professional Nurse Wallchart. MacMillan Magazines

Boston Consulting Group (2005) Growth strategy for ostomy care. In: Herlufson P, Olsen AG, Carlsen B, *et al* (2006) Study of peristomal skin disorders in patients with permanent stomas. *Br J Nurs* **15**(16): 854–62

Collett K (2002) Practical aspects of stoma management. *Nurs Standard* **17**(8): 45–52

Department of Health (2005) *Consultation Document on the Arrangements for Paying Appliance Contractors*. Available online at: www.dh.gov.uk/en/Consultation/Closedconsultations/DH_4072797 (last accessed 6 September 2007)

Faithful S (2001) Radiotherapy. In: J Corner, C Bailey, eds. *Cancer Nursing: Care in context*. Blackwell Science, Oxford: 222–61

Fillingham S, Douglas J (1997) *Urological Nursing*. 2nd edn. Baillière Tindall, London

Hall C, Myers C, Phillips RKS (1995) The 554 ileostomy. *Br J Surg* **82**: 1385

Herlufson P, Olsen AG, Carlsen B, *et al* (2006) Study of peristomal skin disorders in patients with permanent stomas. *Br J Nurs* **15**(16): 854–62

IMS Health Incorporated Group (2006) *New Patient Audit*. IMS Hospital Group, London

IMS Health Incorporated Group (2007) *New Patient Audit*. IMS Hospital Group, London

Korinko A, Yurick A (1997) Maintaining skin integrity during radiotherapy. *Am J Nurs* **97**: 40–4

Lawson A (2003) Complications of stomas. In: Elcoat C, ed. *Stoma Care Nursing*. Hollister, London

Lee J (2001) Common stoma problems: a brief guide for community nurses. *Br J Community Nurs* **6**(8): 407–13

Lyon CC, Smith AJ, Griffiths CEM, Beck MH (2000) The spectrum of skin disorders in abdominal stoma patients. *Br J Dermatol* **143**(6): 1248–60

Lyon CC, Beck MH (2001) Irritant reactions and allergy. In: Lyon CC, Smith AJ, ed. *Abdominal Stomas and their Skin Disorders: An atlas of diagnosis and management*. Martin Dunitz Ltd, London

Lyon CC, Smith A (2001) *Abdominal Stomas and their Skin Disorders: An atlas of diagnosis and management*. Martin Dunitz Ltd, London

McGrath A, Fulham J (2005) Understanding chemotherapy and radiotherapy for the individual with a stoma. In: Porrett T, McGarth A, eds. *Stoma Care*. Blackwell Publishing, Oxford

McKenzie FD, Ingram VA (2001) Dansac invent convexity in the management of flush ileostomy. *Br J Nurs* **10**(15): 1005–9

Myers C (1996) *Stoma Care Nursing: A patient-centred approach*. Arnold, London

Nicholls RJ (1996) Surgical procedures. In: Myers C, ed. *Stoma Care Nursing: A patient-centred approach*. Arnold, London

Schuren J, Becker A, Sibbald RG (2005) A liquid film-forming acrylate for peri-wound protection: a systematic review and meta-analysis (3M™ Cavilon™ No Sting Barrier Film). *Int Wound J* **2**(3): 230–8

Shellito P (1998) Complications of abdominal stoma surgery. *Dis Colon Rectum* **41**(12): 1562–72

Smith AJ, Lyon CC, Hart CA (2002) Multidisciplinary care of skin problems in stoma patients. *Br J Nurs* **11**(5): 324–30

Stevens P, James P (2003) Anatomy and physiology associated with stoma care. In: Elcoat C, ed. *Stoma Care Nursing*. Hollister, London

Walsh BA (1992) Urostomy and urinary pH. In: Fillingham S, Douglas J, eds. *Urological Nursing*. 2nd edn. Baillière Tindall, London

Porrett T, McGrath A (2005) *Stoma Care*. Blackwell Publishing, Oxford

Vujnovich A (2004) Peristomal faecal/urine dermatitis and allergy. *Gastrointestinal Nurs* **2**(5): 25–31

Section II: Wound pain and palliative care

CHAPTER 8

PRINCIPLES OF SKIN AND WOUND CARE: THE PALLIATIVE APPROACH

Jane McManus

Patients with advanced illness are at significant risk of skin damage. Cancer patients with cachexia are at particular risk due to their catabolic state, in which the body's subcutaneous fat reserves are depleted, as are patients with reduced oral intake of nutrition and hydration, and those whose mobility is becoming compromised, all of which occur more frequently at the end of life (Langemo *et al*, 2007), and in patients with advanced disease (Naylor, 2005). Langemo and Brown (2006) use the term 'skin failure' to describe the event that occurs when hypoperfusion of the blood vessels in the skin occurs alongside severe dysfunction or failure of other organ systems. As such, pressure ulcers at the end of life may not be preventable or have the ability to be healed (Langemo and Brown, 2006). Other patients may have wounds directly resulting from the disease itself, such as fungating or malignant wounds caused by infiltration of the skin by cancer cells.

One of the challenges in caring for patients with advanced disease is providing holistic nursing care that promotes the integrity of fragile skin, while also attending to other symptoms. For example, a breathless patient may wish to sit up in bed or in a chair to ease the dyspnoea, but this increases pressure and shear forces on the sacrum and heels. A patient in pain may prefer to lie in one particular position, putting this area of skin under prolonged pressure, with likely skin damage. Patient comfort and prevention strategies can be opposing forces in end of life care (Henoch and Gustafsson 2003).

The goals of palliative wound care include reducing pain, odour, exudate, bleeding and infection (McDonald and Lesage, 2006). Some authors have raised concerns with the use of the term 'palliative wound care'. Patients might be labelled 'palliative' if their wounds are too difficult or costly to heal, allowing 'palliative' to excuse poor outcomes (Ennis and Meneses, 2005). However, if the term 'palliative' is used to describe a clinical situation in which the patient's advanced disease and poor prognosis make wound healing an unlikely outcome, it can enlighten decision-making regarding good wound care.

It is important that patient comfort takes priority over preventing skin breakdown and care of the wound in palliative care (Langemo, 2006). However, when wounds and their symptoms worsen following implementation of measures designed to prioritise patient comfort, holding these opposing needs in balance becomes more challenging for clinicians and patients. This chapter will argue that current theories of moist wound management, with healing as the endpoint, are inappropriate for the needs of palliative patients with wounds (Grocott, 2005). It will also describe the principles of skin care, wound management and symptom control with regard to wounds commonly found in patients in the advanced stages of their disease.

Pressure damage to skin at the end of life

Any severely ill patient may develop pressure ulcers. Immobility and prolonged pressure on a body part is the major risk factor, although reduced sensory perception, older age and neurological disability are also important factors (Reifsnyder and Magee, 2005). Dehydration and hypotension compound tissue damage. Further risk factors include general ill health, ischaemic heart disease, peripheral vascular disease, raised body temperature, incontinence and poor nutritional state, especially hypoalbuminaemia and low vitamin and zinc levels (Dealey, 1999). Drugs that suppress sensation, mobility, or blood flow and skin strength are also aggravating factors (McGrath and Breathnach, 2004), such as steroids (Dealey, 1999) and vaso-active drugs often used in cardiac care (Papantonio et al, 1994).

One study of patients receiving home hospice care in the USA highlighted increased incidence of pressure ulcers in patients who had a history of pressure ulcers, were older, had a diagnosis of cancer, central nervous system disorders or dementia and had lower Karnofsky palliative performance scores (Reifsnyder and Magee, 2005).

The occurrence of pressure ulcers varies according to patient group and care setting. The prevalence of pressure ulcers in palliative care ranges from 13–47% (Langemo, 2006). A study in a UK hospice found a 24% prevalence of pressure ulcers (Bale et al, 1995). Research using an audit cycle to reduce pressure ulcer incidence in a UK hospice, found the incidence did not reduce over two years. The author concluded that pressure damage at the end of life may be inevitable (Galvin, 2002). This has been termed 'skin failure' (Langemo and Brown, 2006).

Malignant or fungating wounds

A malignant or fungating wound occurs when tumour invades the epithelium and breaks through the skin surface (Dealey, 1999). The wound may either be ulcerative or proliferative, meaning that the wound forms either ulcerating craters or raised, cauliflower-like nodules (Bridel-Nixon, 1997; Naylor, 2001). Malignant wounds are commonly seen in breast cancer and head/neck cancers (Naylor, 2002). They also occur in cancers of the skin, vulva and bladder (Dealey, 1999). Fungating wounds develop at the site of the primary cancer and also at affected lymph nodes of the axilla and groin (Dealey, 1999). A malignant wound is very unlikely to improve, even if radiotherapy, chemotherapy or surgery offer short-term symptom reduction, because cancer cells continue to grow.

Bridel-Nixon (1997) notes that there is a dearth of published research on fungating wounds. Most articles discuss single cases. The UK incidence and prevalence is difficult to determine, as national cancer registries do not record this information (Thames Cancer Registry, 2005). Few published studies discuss the extent of the problem (Bridel-Nixon, 1997). The incidence of malignant wounds in patients with breast cancer appears to be between 2 and 5% (Fairbairn, 1993; Haisfield-Wolfe and Rund, 1997; Grocott, 1999). A 10-year prevalence study at a cancer registry in the USA revealed that 367 (5%) of 7316 patients had cutaneous malignancies, of which 38 had wounds resulting from direct local invasion, 337 had metastatic wounds, and eight had both (Lookingbill *et al*, 1990). Malignant wounds affect a small group of people, but provide major challenges that will be discussed.

How fungating wounds develop and the problems they generate is determined by a combination of factors. As cancerous cells multiply, blood and lymph vessels distort, affecting the flow of blood and lymph. This disrupts haemostasis, alters lymphatic, interstitial and cellular environments, causing tissue hypoxia and necrosis. This encourages infection by organisms that thrive in dead tissue. Eventually, blood vessels may be eroded by tumour, causing bleeding (Bridel-Nixon, 1997).

Wound management theories

Modern wound healing theory developed from the work of Winter (1962, 1963). Winter (1962) examined the rate of epithelialisation in experimental wounds cut into the skin of healthy pigs, comparing wounds with a natural scab exposed to the air against wounds that were covered with polythene film. He found that epithelialisation occurred more quickly in the latter. In exposed wounds, epidermal cells migrated from hair follicles and the wound edges, whereas, in covered wounds, epidermal cells migrated through serous exudate, forming a new epidermal layer above the dermis (Winter, 1962).

The principle of moist wound healing led to the development of the first 'scientific' wound dressings to support optimal healing processes, that have revolutionised wound management (Benbow, 2005). These products include hydrogels to retain/bring moisture to the wound, hydrocolloids to absorb small amounts of excess moisture without drying the wound bed, absorbent foams, alginates, adhesive dressings, non-adhesive dressings and silicone-based low adherent dressings.

Winter's (1962) research focused only on acute, superficial wounds, but the results have been used to generate a theory of moist wound healing for all types of wounds of varying aetiologies. Moist wound healing has become the gold standard of current clinical care and product development. However, the theory of moist wound healing does not provide a basis for satisfactory management of every wound seen in palliative care practice.

While a moist environment at the wound site has been shown to aid the rate of epithelialisation in superficial wounds (Eaglstein *et al*, 1988; Agren *et al*, 2001; Parnham, 2002), excess moisture at the wound site also causes maceration of the periwound skin (Cutting and White, 2002). It is clear that wounds need a balanced level of moisture to heal.

Another contemporary approach to wound healing is 'wound bed preparation'. This involves priming the wound to create optimal conditions for healing and removing factors that impede healing such as necrotic tissue, infection and exudate (Falanga, 2000).

Principles of wound bed preparation

Necrotic tissue needs to be removed (debrided) from the wound. This occurs naturally (autolysis), conducted by phagocytic cells in the wound bed, but can be accelerated by the use of enzymes, sterile maggots, Manuka honey or surgical techniques that cut away dead tissue (Romanelli and Mastronicola, 2002). Historically, debridement was considered a treatment to be given once for each wound, unless more necrotic tissue formed. Following debridement, the wound would be expected to heal (Dealey, 1999). However, in chronic wounds, where the healing process has faltered, necrotic tissue may recur. The acute wound debridement model must be tailored to fit chronic wound pathophysiology. Repeated debridement of necrotic tissue is likely to be necessary and has been termed 'maintenance debridement' (Falanga, 2000).

The damaging properties of chronic wound exudate have already been outlined. Managing exudate is a fundamental principle of wound bed preparation. However, containing large volumes of fluid in an effective, reliable and acceptable wound dressing over a wide variety of body locations remains an unmet challenge for dressing manufacturers (Grocott, 2000).

A more recent concept of moist wound healing is 'moisture balance' (Bishop *et al*, 2003). This theory proposes that a balance must be struck between excessive wound fluid, particularly in chronic wounds, which can cause maceration of the periwound skin destroying some of the beneficial processes occurring in the wound, and a wound surface exposed to air which then forms a dry, hard scab that can delay healing (Winter and Scales, 1963). Despite the vast amounts of research undertaken, the optimal level of wound exudate allowing healing remains unestablished (Cutting, 1999).

Bishop *et al* (2003) propose that wound dressings need to be designed for moisture balance. Dressings must absorb and contain exudate away from the wound surface, while ensuring that the wound surface remains moist. These components should be available as a single dressing or a simple dressing system that is secure and effective. This theory and the associated features of dressings designed for exuding chronic wounds, is appropriate where the wound has the potential for healing. However, in situations where healing is unlikely, such as malignant wounds and in patients with a short prognosis, the exudate needs to be managed in such a way that causes minimal impact upon the patient. If the wound surface can be dried to slow the rate and volume of exudate produced, some reduction of the discomfort and distress associated with very wet wounds may be achieved.

Dry wound management: an alternative to moist wound healing in palliative care?

In palliative wound care, a wound that is maintained with a dry scab, preventing the wound bed underneath from producing large volumes of exudate (Winter and Scales, 1963), enables a patient with a short prognosis and a non-healing wound to have a wound managed without a complex dressing regime to absorb exudate, prevent maceration, odour and infection. If it were possible for patients who have dry wounds to have the dry scab maintained and protected without a dressing that creates a moist wound environment, dry wound management would be a viable alternative in palliative wound care. Goals of chronic wound management at the end of life need to shift towards relieving suffering, maintaining function and enabling the patient to engage in activities that are important to them (Enoch and Price, 2004). This requires research to determine how palliative wounds can be managed to fulfil these goals without using healing as the endpoint of research study.

There has been some interest in scabs that form naturally on exposed wounds. There is a need to investigate their properties to understand their role in wound healing and how that may be integrated into current wound management research (Nelson, 1995).

Alternative endpoints in palliative care

The goals in palliative care of symptom control and psychosocial support can be transferred into wound care for palliative patients whose wounds will not heal. This concept of a stable, non-healing wound as a goal of care is relatively new (Ennis, 2001). However, it is important that, if healing stops being the goal and 'palliative wound care' becomes the focus, that palliation follows careful, holistic assessment of the wound and patient, so that it does not become the easier or cheaper option for resource-poor health services (Ennis and Meneses, 2005). Alternative treatment approaches may prove beneficial to relieve suffering and manage symptoms (Enoch and Price, 2004). Dressing products that are designed to heal acute wounds may not have the same effect on chronic, non-healing wounds (Enoch and Price, 2004).

Factors affecting skin integrity (adapted from Holloway and Jones, 2005):

- drying/dessication through washing
- age and skin type
- environmental/climate/lifestyle and occupation
- nutrition and hydration
- peripheral circulation/oedema
- length of stay in hospital (immobilisation)
- level of consciousness
- trauma
- activity
- faecal/urinary incontinence
- fever/infection
- metabolic state
- immunosuppression
- sensation.

Health problems such as diabetes, underlying skin conditions such as eczema and dermatitis, medications such as corticosteroids may also affect skin integrity (Fore-Pfliger, 2004).

Age-related changes to the skin

The epidermis thins by 50% from the age of 60 (Peters, 2005). The surface between the epidermis and dermis, woven closely together in folds in younger skin, flatten out, increasing the skin's fragility and susceptibility to shearing (Baronowski, 2000). Changes to the collagen in the dermis also occur, making it less elastic and less resilient, and thus looser and more prone to wrinkling (Holloway and Jones, 2005), which again increases the skin's fragility and vulnerability. As the vascularity decreases, it dehydrates more easily; there is also a reduction in sebum and the sense of touch becomes less acute (Desai, 1997)

Concurrent assaults on the ageing skin, such as contact with excess moisture from incontinence (Copson, 2006) or lymphorrhoea (MacLaren, 2001) weaken the fragile skin still further.

Incontinence

It is well-established that maceration of the skin increases the skin's fragility and threatens its integrity, incontinence, both faecal and urinary can cause this damage (Gray *et al*, 2002). Ammonia in urine is caustic to the skin, causing skin irritation and damage (Holloway and Jones, 2005). It also acts as a nutrient for bacteria on the surface of the skin, which multiply (Holloway and Jones, 2005). Pathogenic fungi also grow in the warm, moist environment of incontinence, (Gray *et al*, 2002) and may be present in fiery red, itchy and burning skin rashes (Holloway and Jones, 2005).

Lymphoedema and lymphorrhoea

Lymphoedema is a chronic swelling of the limbs, due to the failure of the lymphatic drainage system to remove protein-rich interstitial fluid from the limb (Hampton and Collins, 2004). The lymphatic system is a network of vessels in the dermis, similar to blood vessels, carrying lymphatic fluid from the interstitial system to the blood stream via lymphatic channels and trunks (MacLaren, 2001). The management of lymphoedema, to reduce the volume of misplaced lymph fluid and prevent skin breakdown, involves a four-step process, according to the British Lymphology Society (BLS) (Mortimer, 1997):

* skin care advice
* appropriate advice regarding exercise
* external compression or support
* simple lymphatic drainage massage for individuals to use themselves.

It is beyond the scope of this chapter to discuss lymphoedema management in detail, however, the prevention and management of lymphorrhoea are challenging problems in end of life skin care and will be outlined.

If a limb becomes filled with sufficient lymphoedema that the skin is stretched taut, there is a significant risk of skin breaks, allowing some of the lymphatic fluid to leak out through the broken skin surface. This can lead to damage to the surrounding skin in the form of skin maceration and further breakdown, and the break in the skin's outer layer provides a vehicle for infection to enter the body (Ling *et al*, 1997). The principle aims when treating lymphorrhoea are to cover the site of the break to reduce the risk of infection, notwithstanding the fragility of the skin in a lymphoedematous limb, and gentle compression bandaging to reduce the volume of fluid leaking from the skin break (MacLaren, 2001). For some patients, the discomfort associated with compression bandaging may be too much, and a supportive bandage over absorbent dressings, which are changed as often as required to prevent maceration, may be more appropriate.

Providing good skin care

At St Christopher's Hospice, a Good Skin Care Guidance (St Christopher's Hospice Skin and Wound Group, 2006) has been developed from clinical and research experience in end of life care, which has three cornerstones: assessment, cleansing and pressure reduction.

Assessment

The National Institute for Clinical Excellence (NICE) guidelines (NICE, 2003) recommend that assessment of the skin should include an assessment of the following signs:

- persistent erythema
- non-blanching erythema
- blisters
- discolouration
- localised heat
- localised oedema and localised induration (firmness of the soft tissues due to inflammation).

If the erythema blanches (turns white) with light finger pressure, the microcirculation is intact, although the redness has been caused by a rush of arterial blood (hyperaemia) flowing to an area of skin that has been subjected to pressure (Scanlon and Stubbs, 2004). However, if the erythema does not blanche, the microcirculation has been damaged due to the intensity or duration of pressure, which is known as non-blanching erythema or hyperaemia, and is classified as a stage 1 pressure ulcer in most classification systems (Bethnell, 2003).

Although looking for signs of erythema may be appropriate for patients with pale skin, in darkly pigmented skin redness will not be apparent as an early indicator of skin damage (Scanlon and Stubbs, 2004). In this instance, the NICE guidelines (2003) recommend looking out for the following signs:

- purplish/bluish localised areas of skin
- localised heat that, if tissue becomes damaged, is replaced by coolness
- localised oedema and localised induration.

Associated with the erythema are other changes due to the inflammatory reaction that occurs when the tissue is damaged. These include localised oedema, heat and pain. If the damage has caused necrosis of local tissues, the area may feel cool, and there may be a bluish tinge to the skin. If the damage occurred to an area of soft tissue, the area may feel firm (indurated) due to the oedema (Scanlon and Stubbs, 2004).

The St Christopher's guidance suggests conducting a pressure ulcer risk assessment on admission, which is reviewed weekly and as the patient's overall condition changes. The skin should be visually inspected at every episode of care, and the results and ensuing care requirements documented in the notes.

Skin cleansing

The use of soap and water in the frequent cleansing of a patient's skin leads to dryness and decreases the skin integrity by (Dealey, 1995):

- increasing the skin's pH (Kirsner and Froelich, 1998), encouraging bacteria that prefer an alkaline environment (Voegeli, 2005)
- removing sebum and natural moisturising factors from the skin surface (Peters, 2001), making the skin more vulnerable to damage from fluids, shear and friction (Peters, 2005)
- the presence of soap residues left on the skin after washing, and the possibility of chemical irritation through the use of perfumed soaps (Kirsner and Froelich, 1998)
- friction damage from repeated drying of the skin after cleansing.

Incontinence dermatitis from repeated skin contact with body fluids further harms the skin, making it even more susceptible to friction. Guidance from both the European Pressure Ulcer Advisory Panel (EPUAP, 1998) and NICE (2003) have acknowledged the importance of skin care in pressure ulcer prevention.

There have been several studies into the use of skin care protocols involving specific skin cleansing agents, barrier creams and films (Bale *et al*, 2004; Cole and Nisbet, 2004). These studies have all demonstrated the benefits of skin cleansers that are not soap-based, alongside protective barrier creams or films, in the protection of vulnerable skin and the prevention of pressure damage.

The St Christopher's skin cleansing guidance incorporates earlier work at the hospice into the advantages of an emollient, Diprobase® (Schering-Plough), as a skin-cleansing and moisturising agent rather than soap and other moisturising creams. Diprobase cream is an emollient containing white soft paraffin, cetostearyl alcohol (emulsifying agent), liquid paraffin, cetomacrogol (emulsifying agent) and chlorocresol (antimicrobial preservative). It feels greasy on application to the skin, but is easily absorbed and provides an oily layer over the epidermis to reduce evaporation of water from the skin.

It is used in the hospice as a cleansing cream (dispersing it in washing water by applying some to a disposable dry cloth which is wrung out in the water to create a milky effect), as well as a moisturiser for skin. Two or three drops of essential oil can be added as a fragrance if the patient chooses. It is well-tolerated by most patients, although it contains alcohol which is known to be an irritant to some people's skin (Peters, 2005).

As a barrier product between the skin and the irritant, such as urine or faeces, Cavilon™ Durable Barrier Cream (3M) is recommended in small amounts on skin in contact with moisture such as urine or faeces. Over-application of these products may reduce the effectiveness of incontinence pads by clogging or interfering with their absorbency (Williams, 2001). If the skin is broken, Cavilon™ No Sting Barrier Film is used instead. Cavilon™ can last up to 72 hours (Williams, 1998), but this is dependent on the frequency of skin cleansing that is required by the patient.

This guidance has standardised patient hygiene care, and there is anecdotal evidence that patient skin integrity has improved since the introduction of the guidance, although a formal evaluation has not yet been conducted.

Pressure reduction

Although some practitioners recommend turning vulnerable patients every two hours (Langemo *et al*, 2007), the NICE guidance for pressure ulcer prevention (2003) recommends that the frequency of repositioning should be determined by the results of skin inspection and individual needs rather than by a ritualistic schedule. At the end of life, the patient's symptoms, such as nausea or pain may make effective repositioning difficult (Langemo, 2006; Langemo *et al*, 2007), although efforts should still be made to minimise skin damage to vulnerable areas of the body such as the heels by using a pillow or heel protectors to elevate them.

Some patients will refuse to be turned, and while this may pose a challenge to those caring for them, the patient's wishes should be explored and respected.

The St Christopher's Hospice Guidance suggests that patients should be repositioned regularly, not only to reduce pressure damage, but also to maintain movement in joints, prevent contractures and for psychosocial reasons. The positions should be safe, suitable for the individual and their condition, reduce pressure generally or on areas at particular risk, be comfortable and acceptable to the individual and allow for meals, rest periods, treatments and visitors. The frequency of position change will be based on assessment of risk, the general condition of the patient, and the equipment being used.

Symptom control in end of life wound care

The presence of a wound has consequences for the patient, their family and healthcare providers. There are also financial consequences of managing a wound.

Wounds occur in some patients as one of the consequences of advanced disease of all aetiologies. Studies have assessed the symptoms experienced by patients in the last year of life and wounds contribute to a significant number of these symptoms. One well-known study is the Regional Study of Care for the Dying, which found that 28% of dying people had 'bedsores' in the last year of life, and for 55% of those patients, they were 'very distressing' (Addington-Hall and McCarthy, 1995).

In a Danish qualitative study into the impact of malignant breast wounds on femininity, sexuality, emotions and feelings of 12 women with advanced breast cancer, the wounds and symptoms of malodour and exudate caused the women to feel less feminine and less self-confident (Lund-Nielson *et al*, 2005).

When wounds in palliative care are assessed, the assessment should include psychological assessment of the patient and their family. Care must focus on the maximisation of coping strategies. These patients often express their needs as fears (Langemo, 2006).

Exudate

When the skin is injured causing a wound, fluid accumulates more readily in the wounded tissues. Histamine is released from wounded cells causing plasma to leak from blood vessels, resulting in local oedema (Thomas, 1997). It becomes more difficult for interstitial fluid pressure to be maintained, affecting the control of fluid in blood and lymph systems (Bishop *et al*, 2003). Granulation tissue, which may be present in the wound, can absorb more water than normal skin tissue, also increasing tissue fluid accumulation at the wound site.

Inflammation, which occurs as part of the post-injury process, results in dilation of capillaries increasing their permeability to fluid (Dealey, 1999). An excess of leaking fluid from the wound is known as exudate. It is normally a pale, straw-coloured, watery fluid, which becomes more viscous and opaque because of leukocytes, albumin, macrophages and cell debris (Cutting and White, 2002).

Exudate volume has traditionally been described using subjective terms of light, moderate or heavy (Cutting, 1999). This subjectivity may hinder appropriate dressing selection, as imprecise assessments will result in dressings being chosen on a 'best guess' basis. Dressings that are inappropriately selected, may not perform as effectively as they should.

The nature of acute wound exudate has been found to be substantially different to that of chronic wound exudate. The difference lies predominantly in the presence of tissue-destructive enzymes (proteinases) in the latter (Trengrove *et al*, 1999). These proteinases serve a useful purpose in wound healing in small amounts (Bishop *et al*, 2003), but damage chronic wounds and their surrounding skin (Barrick *et al*, 1999). They contribute directly to chronic wound enlargement (Cutting and White, 2002). Periwound skin is known to be at increased risk of damage compared to healthy skin as it is affected by tissue inflammation (Walker *et al*, 1997). Chronic wound exudate poses serious problems.

There is a growing body of research evidence suggesting that it is not excessive fluid at the wound *per se* that causes healing problems and maceration, but rather the nature of the fluid and its components that cause problems (Bishop *et al*, 2003). Breuing *et al* (1992) used special 'wound chambers' on the skin to maintain a wet environment on the wound using saline, demonstrating that healing was unimpaired and possibly improved, with no maceration and reduced scarring, compared with uncovered wounds. Other work has shown that moist or wet wounds heal as effectively as each other compared with a dry environment (Vogt *et al*, 1995), so long as the composition of the fluid is not detrimental to the wound itself.

This use of moist wound healing theories can be problematic in some clinical situations, in particular, wounds that are being managed at the end of life and are not going to heal, where the volume of moisture produced by the wound is absorbed with varying success by dressing products. In patients with advanced disease who develop wounds, healing is often unrealistic. For these patients, the moist wound environment may be a disadvantage. The moisture must be contained using dressing products, which provide a good fit that does not leak (Grocott, 2000). Dressings require regular reapplication. The serous fluid, proteins and sugars present in the moist wound provide a growing medium for microbes that compound the difficulties of managing non-healing wounds.

Odour

Malodorous wounds can be very distressing for the patient. Patients' relationships may be affected (Douglas, 2001; Lund-Nielsen *et al*, 2005), contributing to social isolation (Douglas, 2001; Naylor, 2002). Wound odour is produced by bacteria that are present in necrotic tissue of the wound (McDonald and Lesage, 2006). In a wound that is expected to heal, debridement of the necrotic tissue is a priority (McDonald and Lesage 2006). In fungating wounds, debridement must be done carefully using non-surgical techniques, as the wounds are likely to be friable and have a tendency to bleed (Naylor, 2002). The use of systemic and topical antibiotics (McDonald and Lesage, 2006), as well as silver dressings as antimicrobials, charcoal dressings to bind the odour molecules, and topical honey (Naylor, 2002), may assist in the management of odour. Any creams or ointments applied topically may increase the volume of exudate produced, which may cause further wound management problems.

Infection

Not all chronic wounds will be infected with micro-organisms, but they will all contain microbes. The point at which microbial colonisation becomes problematic for the wound depends on the numbers and virulence of the microbes and the extent of the immune response triggered (Cutting and Harding, 1994). There are four categories of microbial presence in a wound: contamination, colonisation, critical colonisation and infection. Infection of a chronic wound produces an enhanced and prolonged inflammatory response (Romanelli and Mastronicola, 2002). This causes more damage to the wound and reduces the immune response of the patient (Dow and Ronald, 1994). This masks some of the symptoms of chronic wound infection (Romanelli and Mastronicola, 2002), making the presence of infection less obvious and, therefore, less likely to be investigated, diagnosed and treated.

A recently discovered element of chronic wound infection is 'biofilm' (Sibbald *et al*, 2000; *Chapter 12*). Bacteria exist in wounds in microcolonies, which attach to the wound bed and secrete a biochemical liquid that helps to protect them from antiseptics and antibiotics (Davey and O'Toole, 2000).

The presence of infection or critical colonisation will prevent a wound from healing (Romanelli and Mastronicola, 2002); therefore, reducing microbial numbers to minimise their impact is an important component of encouraging a chronic wound to heal. Additionally, symptoms of odour, exudate and pain can be reduced if the microbial cause is treated (Naylor, 2005).

Pain

Many patients with pressure ulcers experience moderate to severe pain during wound care, dressing changes and debridement. Dressing removal is often the most painful part of the wound management regime (Langemo, 2006). Analgesia should be given systemically or topically before the dressing procedure (Naylor, 2001). Sensitive psychological care, ie. relaxation, music, distraction and gentle conversation may also help pain management (Langemo, 2006). Pain is limited by the use of dressings that are minimally traumatic to remove and cleansing of the wound by gentle irrigation with warmed normal saline (Langemo, 2006). There is a lack of data about the pain experienced by patients with fungating wounds, although one small study (n=13) found that 38% of paitents with fungating wounds experienced pain (Haisfield-Wolfe and Baxendale-Cox, 1999).

There is a growing body of research to suggest that open wounds that are painful may respond to the application of topical opioids such as morphine (Twillman *et al*, 1999) or diamorphine (Back and Findlay, 1995) in a carrying hydrogel. The underpinning theory concerns opioid receptors on sensory nerve endings in the peripheral nervous system (Twillman *et al*, 1999), which are stimulated in the presence of the wound and associated inflammation.

Dressing fit problems

Dressings that have been developed in response to Winter's (1962, 1963) theory maintain moist conditions by ensuring low moisture-vapour loss from the wound. They tend to have a poor capacity to manage large volumes of exudate satisfactorily. They exhibit problems with fit and fixation to a moving body (Grocott, 2000). It has been argued that a radical revision of dressing products in terms of size, presentation, thickness of materials and fixation methods is needed in the light of substantial case study evidence of exuding wounds in palliative care (Grocott, 2000; Seaman, 2006). Evidence from dressing research for heavily exuding wounds demonstrates the benefits of a two-layer dressing system, with the primary contact layer drawing exudate from the wound into a secondary absorbent layer (Grocott, 2000).

Conclusion

Wounds are a symptom of advanced disease, as demonstrated in symptom prevalence studies in palliative care. Chronic wounds in palliative care are mainly of the pressure ulcer and malignant type. Modern wound healing theory developed from the work of Winter (1962, 1963) who demonstrated faster epithelialisation in superficial pig wounds. Winter's theory has been translated to the management of all wounds at all stages of healing. Moist wound healing is the gold standard of current clinical care and product development. Two theories have evolved from moist wound healing: wound bed preparation and moisture balance.

While the prevention of skin damage due to pressure, friction or incontinence should be the primary goal, it is inevitable that some patients will experience a break in their skin integrity at the end of life (Naylor, 2005; Langemo, 2006). Lymphoedema, which may accompany advanced cancer, affecting either the lower or upper limbs also causes skin problems, especially when the limb swelling results in lymphorrhoea. Good skin care is paramount when caring for patients at the end of life, as damage to their fragile skin is easy to cause and challenging to heal.

The nursing skills required for end of life wound care are to prevent the occurrence of damage where possible, minimise the worsening of any wounds that occur by employing an effective wound care regime, attending at all times to the physical symptoms and psychological needs of the patient, and providing reassurance and explanations to those who are alongside the patient that while 'skin failure' can occur at the end of life (Langemo, 2006) despite good skin care, its effects will be managed as effectively as possible to minimise its impact.

Effective palliative wound care relies on attention to maceration, friction and shear forces, nutrition and hydration, as well as a focus on patient mobility and the support surfaces they are nursed on, although the relative risks of each factor are not known. Evidence shows that the effects of chronic wounds are physical (exudate, malodour, infection, pain and dressing fit problems), psychological, emotional and social. In end of life care, alternative surrogate or intermediate endpoints, rather than wound healing, may be appropriate goals, with patient comfort and choice being key to success.

References

Addington-Hall J, McCarthy M (1995) Dying from cancer: results of a national population-based investigation. *Palliative Med* 9(4): 295–305

Agren MS, Karlsmark T, Hansen JB, Rygaard J (2001) Occlusion versus air exposure on full-thickness biopsy wounds. *J Wound Care* 10(8): 301–4

Back IN, Findlay I (1995) Analgesic effect of topical opioids on painful skin ulcers. *J Pain Symptom Management* 10: 493.

Bale S, Finlay I, Harding KG (1995) Pressure sore prevention in a hospice. *J Wound Care* 4(10): 465–8

Bale S, Tebble N, Jones V, Price P (2004) The benefits of implementing a new skin care protocol in nursing homes. *J Tissue Viability* 14(2):44–50

Baranowski S (2000) Skin tears: the enemy of frail skin. *Adv Skin Wound Care* 13(3): 123–6

Barrick B, Campbell EJ, Owen CA (1999) Leukocyte proteinases in wound healing: roles in physiologic and pathologic processes. *Wound Rep Regen* 7(6): 410–22

Benbow M (2005) *Evidence-based Wound Management*. Whurr Publishers, London

Bethnell E (2003) Controversies in classifying and assessing grade 1 pressure ulcers. *J Wound Care* **12**(1): 33–6

Bishop SM, Walker M, Rogers AA, Chen WY (2003) Importance of moisture balance at the wound-dressing interface. *J Wound Care* **12**(4): 125–8

Breuing K, Eriksson E, Liu P, Miller DR (1992) Healing of partial thickness porcine skin wounds in a liquid environment. *J Surg Res* **52**(1): 50–8

Bridel-Nixon J (1997) Other chronic wounds. In: Morison M, Moffatt C, Bridel-Nixon J, Bale S, eds. *The Nursing Management of Chronic Wounds.* 2nd edn. Mosby, London: 221–44

Cole L, Nisbet C (2004) A three-year multi-phase pressure ulcer prevalence/incidence study in a regional referral hospital. *Ostomy/Wound Management* **50**(11): 33–40

Copson D (2006) Management of tissue excoriation in older patients with urinary or faecal incontinence. *Nurs Standard* **21**(7): 57–66

Cutting KF (1999) The causes and prevention of maceration of the skin. *J Wound Care* **8**(4): 200–1

Cutting KF, Harding KG (1994) Criteria for identifying wound infection. *J Wound Care* **3**(4): 198–201

Cutting KF, White RJ (2002) Maceration of the skin and wound bed. 1: Its nature and causes. *J Wound Care* **11**(7): 275–8

Davey ME, O'Toole GA (2000) Microbial biofilms: from ecology to molecular genetics. *Microbiol Mol Biol Rev* **64**(4): 847–67

Dealey C (1995) Pressure sores and incontinence: a study evaluating the use of topical agents in skin care. *J Wound Care* **4**(3): 103–5

Dealey C, ed (1999) *The Care of Wounds: A Guide for Nurses.* 2nd edn. Blackwell Science, London

Desai H (1997) Ageing and wounds. Part 2: healing in old age. *J Wound Care* **6**(5): 237–9

Douglas V (2001) Living with a chronic leg ulcer: an insight into patients' experiences and feelings. *J Wound Care* **10**(9): 355–60

Dow G, Ronald A (1994) Skin tests. In: Hoeprich P, Jordan M, Ronald A, eds. *Infectious Diseases: treatise of infectious processes.* JB Lippincott, Philadelphia

Eaglstein WH, Davis SC, Mehle AL, Mertz PM (1988) Optimal use of an occlusive dressing to enhance healing. Effect of delayed application and early removal on wound healing. *Arch Dermatol* **124**(3): 392–5

Ennis WJ (2001) Healing: can we? Must we? Should we? *Ostomy/Wound Management* **47**(9): 6–8

Ennis WJ, Meneses P (2005) Palliative care and wound care: two emerging fields with similar needs for outcome data. *Wounds* **17**(4): 99–104

Enoch S, Price P (2004) Should alternative endpoints be considered to evaluate outcomes in chronic recalcitrant wounds? World Wide Wounds. Available online at: www.worldwidewounds.com/2004/october/Enoch-Part2/Alternative-Endpoints-To-Healing.html (last accessed 2 March, 2007)

European Pressure Ulcer Advisory Panel (1998) *Pressure ulcer prevention guidelines*. EPUAP, Oxford

Fairbairn K (1993) Towards better care for women: understanding fungating breast lesions. *Prof Nurse* 9(3): 204–8

Falanga V (2000) Classifications for wound bed preparation and stimulation of chronic wounds. *Wound Rep Regen* 8(5): 347–52

Fore-Pfliger J (2004) The epidermal skin barrier: implications for the wound care practitioner, part II. *Adv Skin Wound Care* 17(9): 480–8

Galvin J (2002) An audit of pressure ulcer incidence in a palliative care setting. *Int J Palliative Nurs* 8(5): 214–21

Gray M, Ratliff C, Donovan A (2002) Perineal skin care for the incontinent patient. *Adv Skin Wound Care* 15(4): 170–8

Grocott P (1999) The management of fungating wounds. *J Wound Care* 8(5): 232–4

Grocott P (2000) The palliative management of fungating malignant wounds. *J Wound Care* 9(1): 4–9

Grocott P (2005) Commentary: A guide to wound management in palliative care. *Int J Palliative Nurs* 11(11): 579

Haisfield-Wolfe ME, Baxendale-Cox LM (1999) Staging of malignant cutaneous wounds: a pilot study. *Oncol Nurs Forum* 26(6): 1055–64

Haisfield-Wolfe ME, Rund C (1997) Malignant cutaneous wounds: a management protocol. *Ostomy/Wound Management* 43(1): 56–66

Hampton S, Collins F (2004) Assessment, management and treatment of leg and foot ulceration. In: *Tissue Viability*. Whurr Publishers Ltd, London: chap 5

Henoch I, Gustafsson M (2003) Pressure ulcers in palliative care: development of a hospice pressure ulcer risk assessment scale. *Int J Palliative Nurs* 9(11): 474–84

Holloway S, Jones V (2005) The importance of skin care and assessment. *Br J Nurs* 14(22): 1172–76

Kirsner RS, Froelich CW (1998) Soaps and detergents: understanding their composition and effect. *Ostomy/Wound Management* 44(3A): 62–70

Langemo DK (2006) When the goal is palliative. *Adv Skin Wound Care* 19: 148, 150–4

Langemo DK, Brown G (2006) Skin fails too: acute, chronic and end-stage skin failure. *Adv Skin Wound Care* 19: 206–11

Langemo D, Anderson J, Hanson D, Thompson P, Hunter S (2007) Understanding palliative wound care. *Nursing* 37(1): 65–66

Ling J, Duncan A, Laverty D, Hardy J (1997) Lymphorrhoea in palliative care. *Eur J Palliative Care* 4: 50–2

Lookingbill DP, Spangler N, Sexton FM (1990) Skin involvement as the presenting sign of internal carcinoma. A retrospective study of 7316 cancer patients. *J Am Acad Dermatol* 22(1): 19–26

Lund-Nielsen B, Muller K, Adamsen L (2005) Malignant wounds in women with breast cancer: feminine and sexual perspectives. *J Clin Nurs* 14(1): 56–64

MacLaren J-A (2001) Skin changes in lymphoedema: pathophysiology and management options. *Int J Palliative Nurs* 7(8): 381–8

McDonald A, Lesage P (2006) Palliative management of pressure ulcers and malignant wounds in patients with advanced illness. *J Palliative Med* 9(2): 285–95

McGrath JA, Breathnach SM (2004) Wound healing. In: Burns T, Breathnach S, Cox N, Griffiths C, eds. *Rook's Textbook of Dermatology*. 7th edn. Blackwell Science, Oxford

Mortimer PS (1997) *British Lymphology Society Strategy for Lymphoedema Care*. British Lymphology Society, Caterham

Naylor W (2001) Assessment and management of pain in fungating wounds. *Br J Nurs* 10(22; Suppl): S33–S40

Naylor W (2002) Malignant wounds: aetiology and principles of management. *Nurs Standard* 16(52): 45–53

Naylor W (2005) A guide to wound management in palliative care. *Int J Palliative Nurs* 11(11): 572–9

Nelson EA (1995) Moist wound healing: critique II. *J Wound Care* 4: 370–1

National Institute for Clinical Excellence (2003) *Pressure Ulcer Prevention. Clinical Guideline 7*. NICE, London

Papantonio CT, Wallop JM, Kolodner KB (1994) Sacral ulcers following cardiac surgery: incidence and risks. *Adv Wound Care* 7(2): 24–36

Parnham A (2002) Moist wound healing: does the theory apply to chronic wounds? *J Wound Care* 11(4): 143–6

Peters J (2001) Caring for dry and damaged skin in the community. *Br J Community Nurs* 6(12): 645–51

Peters J (2005) Exploring the use of emollient therapy in dermatological nursing. *Br J Nurs* 14(9): 494–502

Reifsnyder J, Magee H (2005) Development of pressure ulcers in patients receiving home hospice care. *Wounds* 17(4): 74–9

Romanelli M, Mastronicola D (2002) The role of wound-bed preparation in managing chronic pressure ulcers. *J Wound Care* 11(8): 305–10

Scanlon E, Stubbs N (2004) Pressure ulcer risk assessment in patients with darkly pigmented skin. *Prof Nurse* 19(6): 339–41

Seaman S (2006) Management of malignant fungating wounds in advanced cancer. *Semin Oncol Nurs* 22(3): 185–93

Sibbald RG, Williamson D, Orsted HL, Campbell K, Keast D, Krasner D, Sibbald D (2000) Preparing the wound bed — debridement, bacterial balance and moisture balance. *Ostomy/Wound Management* 46(11): 14–35

St Christopher's Hospice Skin and Wound Group (2006) *St Christopher's Hospice Clinical Guidance for Skin and Wound Care*. St Christopher's Hospice Skin and Wound Group, St Christopher's Hospice, London

Thames Cancer Registry (2005) *Cancer in South East England 2003*. Thames Cancer Registry, King's College, London

Thomas S (1997) Assessment and management of wound exudate. *J Wound Care* 6(7): 327–30

Trengove NJ, Stacey MC, MacAuley S, *et al* (1999) Analysis of the acute and chronic wound environments: the role of proteases and their inhibitors. *Wound Rep Regen* 7(6): 442–52

Twillman RK, Long TD, Cathers TA, Mueller DW (1999) Treatment of painful skin ulcers with topical opioids. *J Pain Symptom Management* 17(4): 288–92

Voegeli D (2005) Skin hygiene practices, emollient therapy and skin vulnerability. *Nurs Times* 101(4): 57–8

Vogt PM, Andree C, Breuing K, Liu PY, Slama J, Helo G, Eriksson E (1995) Dry, moist and wet skin wound repair. *Ann Plastic Surg* 34(5): 493–9

Walker M, Hulme TA, Rippon MG, Walmsley RS, Gunnigle S, Lewin M, Winsey S (1997) In vitro model(s) for the percutaneous delivery of active tissue repair agents. *J Pharm Sci* 86(12): 1379–84

Williams C (1998) 3M Cavilon No Sting Barrier Film in the protection of vulnerable skin. *Br J Nurs* 7(10): 613–15

Williams C (2001) 3M Cavilon Durable Barrier Cream in skin problem management. *Br J Nurs* 10(7): 469–72

Winter GD (1962) Formation of the scab and the rate of epithelialisation of superficial wounds in the skin of the young domestic pig. *Nature* 193(4812): 293–4

Winter GD (1963) Effect of air exposure and occlusion on experimental human skin wounds. *Nature* 200: 378–9

Winter GD, Scales JT (1963) Effect of air drying and dressings on the surface of a wound. *Nature* 197: 91–2

CHAPTER 9

CANCER AND WOUND CARE

Patricia O'Regan

A diagnosis of cancer and its subsequent treatments gives rise to a set of symptoms and problems that are specific to each individual experiencing the disease trajectory. The nature and severity of these symptoms depends on several factors, including the effect of the disease on the individual, the effect of treatments and the physiological and psychological response.

The intensity of cancer treatments can have major implications in relation to formation of wounds and wound care management. These wounds can lead to problematic long-term care. Cancer itself can give rise to wounds in the form of multiple skin lesions or fungating wounds that frequently have associated symptoms (Naylor *et al*, 2001).

Malignant wounds may occur in up to 5% of patients with cancer and in 10% of patients with metastatic disease (Seaman, 2006).

Cancer treatments and their impact on wound healing

Radiotherapy

Radiotherapy is a localised cancer treatment that is used alone or in conjunction with other treatments such as surgery or chemotherapy. High-energy ionising rays act on cellular DNA, halting cellular replication. The subsequent formation of free radicals then damages healthy tissue, including the skin (Hassey Dow *et al*, 1997). Damage to DNA is repaired by enzymes, with either correction of the damage or fixation of the damage resulting in mutations that can lead to cell dysfunction, inability to proliferate or later carcinogenesis (Dormand _et al_, 2005). The level of damage equates directly with the level of radiation exposure.

Radiotherapy may be administered before surgery to treat undisturbed tissues and to shrink the tumour size, or after surgery to attack cancer cells that may have disseminated beyond the surgical margins. Thus, radiotherapy may be used to cure by eradicating the tumour, to control the growth and spread of disease or to reduce and potentially relieve symptoms of advanced disease. About 60% of all patients with cancer will be treated with radiotherapy at one stage during their disease (Otto, 2001).

As radiotherapy cannot differentiate between normal cells and cancer cells, normal cells within the path of the radiation beam will be affected, causing the patient to experience side-effects (Green and Kinghorn, 1995). Certain tissues are sensitive to radiotherapy, such as the lungs, testes, eyes and ovaries, thus only limited doses of radiotherapy can be given.

Wound healing can be seriously affected by radiotherapy. The long-term effects include skin atrophy, soft tissue fibrosis and microvascular damage, leading to a higher risk of developing problematic, non-healing wounds that are unamenable to surgical repair (Dormand _et al_, 2005).

Clinical manifestations

The response of healthy tissue in the treatment site produces the common side-effects of skin reactions, hair loss and gastrointestinal disturbances (Gates and Fink, 2001). Most of these problems are reversible, except for skin reactions and wound healing where radiotherapy can have long-term detrimental effects. Usually skin reactions occur about two weeks into the course of treatment. They depend on a number of treatment and patient factors, including the patient's age, skin integrity, type of radiation and amount of energy used, chemical and skin irritants used by the patient, nutritional status, presence of skin folds and concurrent chemotherapy (Sitton, 1992). Skin reactions to radiotherapy may be mild, such as dry skin, but may vary from slight erythema to, at its worse, moist desquamation.

Nursing management

Treatment of dry desquamation is similar to erythema. Care of the skin should focus on preventing skin breakdown and relieving the symptoms of burning and itching. The skin should be moisturised daily with an emollient cream. If pruritis and/or pain are present, topical steroid creams and cooled hydrogel sheets should be applied (Naylor *et al*, 2001). Skin folds, moist areas and opposing skin surfaces subject to friction are likely to develop more intense reactions (Gates and Fink, 2001).

The chances of developing a moist skin reaction increases as higher doses of radiotherapy are given. The management of moist desquamation can pose somewhat of a challenge as reactions often develop in awkward places, such as the axilla, neck and perineum, where dressings cannot be easily applied (Faithfull and Wells, 2003). The care of moist desquamation skin reactions is based on the principles of moist wound healing. Management should include:

- wound assessment, including the wound colour, its appearance and the presence of exudate and any signs of infection
- wound management, including irrigation of the wound as well as dressing application.

The type of dressing used is dependent on the amount of exudate present. Common dressings include a hydrogel and a secondary dressing; foam sheets or alginates should be used if bleeding occurs (Naylor *et al*, 2001). Patients may need additional antibiotics if infection and excess exudate are present. Dressings should be changed daily.

The development of moist desquamation may cause many patients to have treatment postponed or completed prematurely. This is not desirable as it may impact on the patient's chances of survival.

Chemotherapy

Chemotherapy is the use of cytotoxic drugs in the treatment of cancer. It is a systemic treatment, rather than localised therapy such as surgery or radiotherapy. Chemotherapy may be used in five ways:

- adjuvant therapy is a course of chemotherapy used in conjunction with other treatments, such as surgery or radiotherapy
- neoadjuvant therapy is chemotherapy given before surgery to shrink the tumour
- primary therapy is the treatment of a localised tumour with only chemotherapy where another form of treatment could also be given

- induction therapy is treatment with chemotherapy where no alternate treatment exists
- combination chemotherapy is the administration of two or more chemotherapy agents.

Chemotherapy drugs affect both normal and malignant cells by altering activity during one or more phases of the cell cycle. Although both types of cells are destroyed by chemotherapy, normal cells have a greater ability to repair and recover than malignant cells. The susceptibility of malignant cells to irreparable damage is used to achieve the therapeutic effect of cytotoxic chemotherapy (Corner and Bailey, 2001).

Chemotherapy is delivered in planned schedules to enable normal cells to recover while killing a number of malignant cells with each administration. It is most effective in frequently dividing cells. Normal body cells with rapid growth changes that are most commonly affected by chemotherapy agents include bone marrow, hair follicles, the mucosal lining of the gastrointestinal tract, the skin and germinal cells (Otto, 2001).

Clinical manifestations

The most common side-effects of chemotherapy drugs include mucositis, nausea and vomiting, skin changes, stomatitis, cardiac toxicity, haematopoietic toxicity (resulting in neutropenia, thrombocytopenia and anaemia), hypersensitive reactions, metabolic alterations, neurotoxicity, ototoxicity, pulmonary toxicity, renal system toxicity, reproductive system dysfunction and fatigue (Otto, 2001).

Chemotherapy can cause significant wound-related problems. Skin reactions associated with chemotherapy include transient erythema, hyperpigmentation, photosensitivity, nail changes and palmar/plantar syndrome.

The administration of specific chemotherapy agents may result in an inflammatory reaction in tissue that has been previously irradiated. This can result in erythema, blisters, hyperpigmentation, oedema, vesicle formation, exfoliation and ulcer formation (Brighton and Wood, 2005). Neutropenia is recognised as being a potential problem for many patients who receive chemotherapy (Kirschbaum, 1998), and is defined as having < 1000 circulating neutrophil cells/mm^2 of blood. Neutropenia results from the destruction of neutrophils by chemotherapeutic agents that cannot distinguish between normal and malignant cells (Fisher *et al*, 1997) and can have grave implications for wound care. Because of a reduction in the number of neutrophils, patients who are neutropenic are at a greater risk of infection and having infected wounds (Kirschbaum, 1998).

Nursing management

Chemotherapy can adversely affect wound healing by inhibiting cell division and protein synthesis. Many chemotherapy drugs can also cause immunosuppression. This can inhibit the inflammatory response in the early stages of wound healing (Lotti *et al*, 1998). Immunosuppressants have a profound negative effect on wound healing by inhibiting the immune response. This reduces the activity of neutrophils and macrophages, thereby increasing the risk of wound infection and delaying the removal of dead tissue and foreign bodies through phagocytosis (Cutting, 1994).

Chemotherapy may decrease the size of a fungating wound by destroying malignant cells and, in turn reducing pressure on nerves and blood or lymph vessels. This can also lessen exudate production and the tendency of the wound to bleed, potentially allowing the wound to heal (Brighton and Wood, 2005).

Chemotherapy causing extravasation and wound-related problems

A number of chemotherapy drugs are known to cause venous irritation. These drugs are known as vesicants. The extravasation of a vesicant drug may cause severe tissue damage that results in the formation of a non-healing necrotic ulcer. Tissue damage may be severe and long term. The tissue damage to the specific area where chemotherapy drug leakage occurs may cause significant pain, cosmetic disfigurement, nerve damage, loss of limb function or even amputation (Stoios, 1999).

Following extravasation of a vesicant drug, tissue ulceration normally forms over a few days, with maximum severity over 2–3 weeks. The degree of tissue damage can be related to several factors, such as amount of drug extravasated, drug concentration, site, needle insertion device and technique. The affected skin tissue appears swollen, tender and red; this can gradually progress to the development of a necrotic ulcer. Ulcers may become wider and deeper over a period of weeks to months and may involve tendons and nerves. Severe necrosis with pain involvement usually indicates the need for surgical intervention (Montrose, 1987).

Surgery

Despite certain limitations, surgery continues to be an important treatment modality for cancer. Surgery has several applications in cancer management and treatment and is often the initial and preferred treatment of choice for many cancers (Moffat and Ketcham, 1994).

Surgical treatment of cancer focuses on five key areas:

- primary treatment involves the removal of a malignant tumour and a margin of adjacent normal tissue
- adjuvant treatment or debulking is the removal of a large tumour burden
- salvage treatment is extensive surgery to treat local recurrence
- palliative treatment involves surgical treatment of related symptoms
- combination treatment combines surgery with other treatment modalities, such as chemotherapy, radiotherapy or immunotherapy (Otto, 2001).

The extent of cancer surgery has changed considerably over the past number of years. Previously, surgery tended to be quite radical involving large surgical excisions, such as mastectomy. Today, surgery tends to be more conservative, such as a lumpectomy followed by further treatment such as radiotherapy. However, major surgery is still necessary in some cases such as those requiring a radical mastectomy. For these patients a wide excision or en bloc dissection is necessary. This involves the removal of the primary tumour, regional lymph nodes, intervening lymphatic channels and involved neighbouring structure (Otto, 2001).

Radical surgery often causes major deformities to the individual as well as loss of function. This can have major psychological implications for the patient as well as a severe impact on body image. This may result in depression and withdrawal from social interactions and normal daily activity. After surgery, patients with cancer often grieve over real or imagined changes in body image or self-worth. Cancer surgeries requiring the largest number of subsequent reconstructive surgeries include the head and neck (facial reconstruction), breast (reconstruction after mastectomy) and superficial tissues (skin graft after resection for melanoma) (Otto, 2001). Reconstructive surgery is carried out with the initial surgery for tumour removal, or following a period of time.

Clinical presentation

As a consequence of the intensity of the surgical treatment, such as a radical mastectomy, many patients develop significant side-effects. These side-effects often result in wounds that are complex and require a well-planned management strategy. Wound-related complications of surgery include:

- haemorrhage and haematoma
- sepsis
- pulmonary complications
- thrombophlebitis
- shock (Corner and Bailey, 2001).

Nursing management

To reduce the risk of cancer wound complications, careful continuous assessment should be carried out on each individual wound.

There are a number of areas that should be focused on, such as:

- wound aetiology — is the wound caused by radiotherapy or is it a fungating wound?
- location, which can affect the rate of healing — is the wound at the site of the radiotherapy field?
- size, depth and shape of wound
- amount and nature of exudate
- is there odour present?
- type of tissue present — is the wound necrotic or sloughy and what specific colour is the wound?
- signs of infection — local and systemic signs such as swelling, heat and redness
- nature and type of pain
- pain related to dressing changes and wound cleansing
- conditions of surrounding skin and episodes of bleeding (Naylor *et al*, 2001).

Advanced cancer and wounds

Fungating wounds

Fungating cancer wounds could be considered the most distressing type of lesion for patients with cancer and, indeed, is the most distressing side-effect of the disease that is most apparent in patients with advanced cancer. These wounds are frequently strongly odorous with exudate that may be serous or blood, which can seep onto clothing and cause extreme distress (Neal, 1991).

Fungating wounds can have a huge negative psychological impact on the individual causing potential withdrawal from social activities and daily life. A fungating wound in a patient with cancer develops from the extension of a malignant tumour into the structure of the skin, producing a raised or ulcerating necrotic lesion (Bennett and Moody, 1995).

Fungating cancer wounds are generally described when malignant tumours infiltrate and erode through the skin. Breast cancer, melanoma, bladder, colon, kidney, ovary, uterus, stomach, head and neck, and lung cancers can all potentially cause fungating wounds (Grocott, 1995), with fungating breast wounds being the most common. Fungating cancer wounds generally occur in older people and in the last six months of life. Patients with cancer can present with a number of symptoms, as fungating cancer lesions generally do not heal. Many of these symptoms can be long term, often persisting until the patient dies.

Clinical presentation

Fungating wounds frequently have many associated symptoms, including: exudate; infection; slough/necrosis; bleeding; pain at wound site; itching and irritation; and malodour (Collinson, 1992). Exudate is considered the most common problem of fungating wounds. Exudate is frequently distressing and embarrassing for the patient, resulting from the common occurrence of leakage onto clothing. The psychological distress caused by a heavy bleed can be devastating to the patient, family and the healthcare professional involved (Naylor *et al*, 2001). It can have devastating effects on the patient's social and personal life, and may result in hospitalisation if the wound tends to bleed heavily.

Nursing management

There has been little research into the incidence and management of fungating cancer wounds. By combining surgery with other treatments, such as chemotherapy, radiotherapy and hormone therapy, mortality rates and disease-free interval rates have increased significantly (Otto, 2001). These treatments may be administered separately or given as a combination. Local treatments include haemostatic agents and topical metronozidole, as well as systemic analgesics, antibiotics or clotting factors, as necessary (Regnard and Tempest, 1992).

The priority in the management of fungating cancer wounds, especially in advanced cancer, should be optimum patient comfort. It may be unnecessary to use dressings that promote optimum conditions for wound healing, as the priority of a dressing should be:

- patient comfort and acceptability
- minimising slough and necrotic tissue
- minimising infection
- containing odour
- containing exudate (Naylor *et al*, 2001).

It is important to select the correct dressing as each type has different absorbent properties. The dressing should have minimal bulk, while preventing leakage and creating an acceptable cosmetic appearance (Thomas, 1997).

Lymphoedema

Lymphoedema is an incurable, progressive condition characterised by chronic swelling, most commonly of a limb and sometimes the adjacent quadrant of the trunk (Corner and Bailey, 2001). Lymphoedema is a frequent complication of cancer and its treatments, and it can have long-term physical implications for the individual.

Lymphoedema is categorised as either primary or secondary, although most patients with cancer develop secondary lymphoedema. Primary lymphoedema is caused by an intrinsic abnormality or insufficiency in the lymphatic system. Secondary lymphoedema occurs because of damage or changes in the lymphatic system resulting from an external cause (Morison *et al*, 2007).

Cancer surgery, radiotherapy and cancer metastasis can produce lymphatic injury that progresses to lymphoedema. Both infection and thrombosis are two common factors that can precipitate lymphoedema in patients who have had surgery and radiotherapy. Other factors that can cause lymphoedema include: postoperative wound complications, including infection/seroma or radiodermatitis; infection of soft tissue of the arm; a tumour on the side of the dormant hand; and obesity (Corner and Bailey, 2001).

Lymphoedema can cause traumatic disfigurement to the patient with cancer, as well as pain and disability. The cancer survivor can be faced with psychological and psychosocial adjustment. Lymphoedema can develop at any time following a diagnosis and/or treatment for cancer and has been reported to occur many years later, especially in the case of breast cancer. Lymphoedema is defined as an oedema of more than three months duration that does not reduce on elevation (Moffatt *et al*, 2003).

Clinical presentation

With the exception of the early stages of lymphoedema (when pitting occurs with the application of pressure and the oedema may be reduced by elevation of the swollen limb), lymphoedema does not reduce significantly with elevation or with diuretic administration (Corner and Bailey, 2001). According to Veitch (1993), skin problems also occur at an early stage as well as in more complicated lymphoedema, including:

- dry skin
- callosites and corns
- fungal infections
- hyperkeratosis
- acute inflammatory episodes (infective and non-infective)
- contact dermatitis.

Nursing management

Treatments are focused on reducing the swelling, minimising complications and teaching the individual to self-care and maintain the improvements in the long term. Treatment is based on compression, exercise, skin care and massage (British Lymphology Society [BLS], 2001a, b).

The components of treatment are combined according to the severity of the condition; whether the individual has no swelling but is known to be at risk of developing lymphoedema, has mild and uncomplicated lymphoedema, has moderate to severe and/or complicated swelling, or has oedema and advanced malignancy (BLS, 2001a, b). Lymphatic massage is a simple form of skin massage used to encourage the movement of lymph along the skin from the swollen congested areas to normally draining areas (Corner and Bailey, 2001).

Manual lymphatic drainage (MLD) is designed to move fluid from swollen areas to those areas of the body where it can naturally drain; a self-massage technique has been developed to enable individuals to maintain and potentially gain further improvement (BLS, 2001a, b). Surgical interventions for lymphoedema are not recommended in patients with cancer, as they have not been proved to be successful in reducing and eradicating the condition.

Skin care is an extremely important component of lymphoedema management and the overall goal of care should be to promote skin integrity and prevent complications from the decreased oxygenation of tissues. The aim of skin care should be to improve the condition of the epidermis and dermis so that they are well hydrated and intact, and to reduce the risk of infection. Skin care should include factors such as: good daily hygiene; regular inspection of the skin; avoiding sources of skin damage such as sun, razors and needles; reducing the risks of cuts and grazes by prompt cleaning; wearing comfortable, loose clothing; daily application of bland emollients (non-perfumed); and the use of specific dermatological products (Corner and Bailey, 2001).

Vulnerable patients

Patients with cancer are in a vulnerable position in that they experience a number of symptoms secondary to their cancer that can have detrimental consequences to effective wound repair and management, as well as to their lives in general. The most frequent and debilitating symptoms include nausea and vomiting, malnutrition/cancer cachexia and fatigue. All of these symptoms can invariably cause problems with nutritional intake and, potentially, malnutrition.

Adequate nutrition is vital for wound healing. However, achieving and maintaining a good nutritional status for patients with cancer is often difficult as 40–80% of all patients with cancer will experience some degree of malnutrition, which is a major cause of morbidity and mortality (Gates and Fink, 2001).

Malnourishment delays wound healing because it reduces collagen synthesis, while plasma proteins essential for effective wound healing may be used elsewhere to satisfy increased energy requirements (Senter and Pringle, 1985). Malnutrition is reported as the cause of death in as many as 20% of patients with cancer (Otto, 2001). Metabolic changes affecting appetite and the use of nutrients cause many patients to lose weight before diagnosis (Ovenson *et al*, 1993).

Cancer treatments, such as surgery, radiotherapy and chemotherapy, can all further reduce food intake because of the development of side-effects such as taste changes, mucositis, pain, nausea and vomiting (Ottery, 1995). Protein-calorie malnutrition (when macronutrient intake cannot meet the body's metabolic needs) is the single most common syndrome resulting from cancer and its treatment. Protein-calorie malnutrition can result in a number of severe and life-threatening symptoms, including progressive weight loss, muscle wasting, skin breakdown, poor wound healing, potential intolerance to therapy, endocrine abnormalities, electrolyte and fluid imbalances and inadequate immune functions (Gates and Fink, 2001).

Despite major progressions in anti-emetics, nausea and vomiting appear to have remained a constant uncomfortable disruptive feature for patients with cancer. People with cancer are at risk of nausea and vomiting from several causes: the cancer treatments (chemotherapy, radiotherapy and surgery, including anaesthesia); progressive disease; and from other factors such as chemicals, central nervous system involvement, and vestibular and visceral effects (Brighton and Wood, 2005). Nausea and vomiting related to chemotherapy occurs in 20–40% of patients, despite the constant use of anti-emetics.

Radiation-induced nausea and vomiting occurs in 10–100% of patients and is dependent on the site of irradiation (Gates and Fink, 2001). The gastrointestinal tract is particularly vulnerable to radiation damage and toxicity occurs when radiotherapy is directed at sites covering the oesophagus, abdomen and pelvis (Faithfull and Wells, 2003). Postoperative nausea and vomiting is a significant feature. Half of patients with advanced cancer experience nausea and vomiting. Sustained nausea and vomiting are associated with anorexia, taste changes, development of food aversions and weight loss with depletion of body stores of protein and fat causing protein-calorie malnutrition (Gates and Fink, 2001). Patients with cancer who are experiencing nausea and vomiting can quite quickly become dehydrated and malnourished. Dehydration also adversely affects optimum wound healing by disturbing cellular metabolism and reducing circulatory blood volume (Naylor *et al*, 2001). Malnourished patients are also at a reduced risk of wound infection because of a reduced immune response (Olde Damink and Soeters, 1997).

Fatigue is the most commonly reported symptom (Winningham *et al*, 1994), and for some patients is the most unpleasant symptom and the most distressing side-effect in connection with cancer and its treatment (Richardson *et al*, 1998). Cancer-related fatigue is a severe problem that is exacerbated by the treatments needed to control and cure the disease. Fatigue has important implications for cancer care as patients may have to discontinue treatments because of it. Also, the doses of some forms of treatment are limited by fatigue.

Patients with cancer have reported fatigue as the symptom that has the most negative impact on their quality of life compared with nausea, depression and pain (the symptoms ranked most highly by oncologists) (Curt *et al*, 2000). Stroemgren *et al* (2002) identified that more than 90% of patients in palliative care suffered from fatigue. Many patients may also become malnourished and anaemic while experiencing chronic fatigue.

Psychological issues

Cancer has a profound psychological impact on patients and their significant others. A diagnosis of cancer can have an immense negative impact on patients and their families. At least 25% of patients develop depression and anxiety, which may lead to a poor quality of life and reduced life expectancy. Patients with cancer are the greatest subgroup of patients who develop depression who have not had a previous history of the illness (Dergotis *et al*, 1988).

Although sadness and a sense of hopelessness may be considered normal reactions to the diagnosis of cancer, other factors can contribute to a depressed mood: the disease process itself; tests, treatments, side-effects and their management; medications; chemotherapy; or a biological depression not necessarily related to the present event. Many people consider a cancer diagnosis as a sentence of impending and painful death. Society still has a collective dread of cancer and considers that cancer means death and pain.

It could be considered that uncertainty is the hallmark of cancer. Throughout their cancer journey, patients are faced with constant uncertainties, such as treatments, side-effects of the cancer and therapies, remission and relapse. Treatment and side-effects as well as the illness itself often necessitate patients with cancer to alter their lifestyle and normal daily living routines. Many patients may lose the ability to work and care for their family, which will then have detrimental effects on all family members.

The psychological impact of a chronic wound varies according to the patient's coping mechanism, the impact on his or her quality of life and the patient's perception of the wound. A fungating wound can have a devastating psychological effect on an individual, especially when it is in an area where it is visible. This could cause the patient to withdraw from society and become isolated. Close relationships may also be severely affected. The sharing of common facilities may cause severe embarrassment, and symptoms such as odour and excessive exudate may lead to a reluctance to go to bed with a partner because of the likelihood of leakage and staining of the patient's clothes or bedding during the night (Naylor *et al*, 2001).

Chronic wounds can severely negatively impact patients' body image, their sense of self-worth and their lives. Caring for a patient with cancer with a chronic wound should encompass an individual, holistic perspective. Assessment and management should involve the psychological, social, emotional and spiritual aspects of the individual patient.

Quality of life issues

According to Krishnassy (2001), when self-perception is altered by the presence of a physical wound, whether this is visible or not, a profound negative association may occur. A person may identify themselves with the malignant wound and consider themselves to be foul, odorous or repulsive. The consequences of living with a malignant wound may also include exudate, infection and bleeding; wound-related pain as well as malodour. Thus, this can have an enormous and detrimental impact on the individual's quality of life, as well as their self esteem. The malignant wound may stop the individual wearing clothes that they desire, thus impacting on their body image and their own personal identity. This could potentially impact on relationships as well as isolating the individual from society.

A common theme to all individuals facing a diagnosis of cancer is the prospect of change and the need for physical, psychological and social adaptation to that change (Perry and Burgess, 2002). The rigorous schedule and the side-effects of surgery, chemotherapy and radiation treatment could interfere significantly with huge aspects of an individual's life such as their diet, lifestyle, sexuality, relationships, financial status, recreation and other activites of daily living that are normally taken for granted. Treatments can be exhausting and could create frustration, irritability, fear and hopelessness.

Completion of treatment can also cause grave anxiety to the individual. Otto (2001) outlines the fact that patients may feel an even greater loss of control when treatment ends than during treatment, due to the fact that they are no longer doing anything to battle cancer. Also, despite the fact that an individual may have received all of their planned treatment successfully, completion can cause patients to feel frightened and vulnerable. Although a disease-free survival may be a reality, this is also a time of uncertainty and ambivalence. After the distraction of dealing with the various aspects of their treatment, this can be a time when people contemplate how to cope with life (Perry and Burgess, 2002). Many patients also find good support mechanisms while attending the hospital/outpatient setting; be it from nursing, medical staff or fellow patients. Completion of treatment also means ceasing these supportive relationships.

The psychological/sociological effect that cancer has on an individual can impact on them for a long period of time, despite the fact that treatment may have been successful. Any changes to their bodily function such as development of fatigue, pain, constipation or nausea may cause grave anxiety and concern. Knowledge of the malignancy process and fear of reoccurrence may incline people to be vigilant of their health status for the rest of their life, often to extreme cases. Otto (2001) highlights that the cancer survivor experiences concerns related to a vast number of areas such as second malignancies, organ dysfunction, fatigue, disability, disfigurement and continuing emotional distress. According to Corner and Bailey (2001), psychological well-being is very much related to physical well-being, so every effort should be made by healthcare professionals to prevent, minimise or treat the physical effects of illness. Enabling patients to feel independent and maintain their own integrity, while at the same time providing support, should be considered to be an important aspect of nursing care.

Conclusion

Cancer causes a great range of distressing and traumatic problems, which are caused by the disease itself and the subsequent treatments. These symptoms or problems are not mutually isolated, but often coexist with other symptoms, having a domino effect on the others, such as the case of nausea/vomiting and anorexia/cachexia. As a result of the necessary intensity of treatments, the impact and severity of symptoms may fluctuate over time throughout the cancer journey.

Many of these symptoms, as well as implications of treatments, have a deleterious effect on wound care management and on the individual. Cancer wounds can result in major irreversible skin damage to the extent of tissue necrosis. They can cause extreme pain and discomfort, which can affect daily activity. They can be disfiguring, foul smelling and appear repulsive to the patient. This can result in an individual's self-esteem, body image and quality of life being severely affected.

Nursing care of the cancer patient with a chronic or fungating wound should not just focus on the physical aspects of care, but encompass communication skills and general advice on how to adapt and promote optimum quality of life.

References

Bennett G, Moody M (1995) *Wound Care for Health Professionals.* Chapman and Hall, London

Brighton D, Wood M (2005) *The Royal Marsden Hospital Handbook of Cancer Chemotherapy.* Churchill Livingstone, London

British Lymphology Society (2001a) *Chronic Oedema Population and Needs.* BLS, Sevenoaks

British Lymphology Society (2001b) *Guidelines for the Use of Manual Lymphatic Drainage and Self-Administered Massage in Lymphoedema.* BLS, Sevenoaks

Collinson G (1992) Improving quality of life in patients with malignant fungating wounds. Second European Conference on Advances in Wound Management Proceedings. In: Naylor W, Laverty D, Mallett J, eds (2001) *The Royal Marsden Hospital Handbook of Wound Management in Cancer Care.* Blackwell Science, Oxford

Corner J, Bailey C (2001) *Cancer Nursing Care in Context.* Blackwell Publishing, Oxford

Curt GA, Breitbart W, Cella D, Groopman JE, Horning SJ, Itri LM, *et al* (2000) Impact of cancer-related fatigue on the lives of patients: new findings from the Fatigue Coalition. *Oncologist* 5: 353–60

Cutting K (1994) Factors affecting wound healing. *Nurs Standard* 8(50): 33–6

Dergotis L, Morrow G, Fetting J, *et al* (1988) The prevalence of psychiatric disorders among cancer patients. *J Am Med Assoc* 249: 751–7

Dormand E, Banwell PE, Goodcare TE (2005) Radiotherapy and wound healing. *Int Wound J* 2(2): 1–20

Faithfull S, Wells M (2003) *Supportive Care in Radiotherapy.* Churchill Livingstone, London

Fisher DS, Knobfm MT, Durivage HJ (1997) *The Cancer Chemotherapy Handbook.* 5th edn. Mosby Inc, Missouri

Gates R, Fink R (2001) *Oncology Nursing Secrets.* 2nd edn. Hanley and Belfus, Philadelphia

Green P, Kinghorn S (1995) Radiotherapy. In: David J, ed. *Cancer Care Prevention, Treatment and Palliation*. Chapman and Hall, London: 113

Grocott P (1995) The palliative management of fungating malignant wounds. *J Wound Care* 4: 240–2

Hassey Dow K, Dunn Bulcholz J, Iwamoto R, *et al* (1997) *Nursing Care in Radiation Oncology*. 2nd edn. WB Saunders, Pennsylvania

Kirschbaum M (1998) Neutropenia: more than a low neutrophil count. *Eur J Oncol Nurs* 2(2): 1, 15–122

Lotti T, Rodofili C, Benci M, *et al* (1998) Wound healing problems associated with cancers. *J Wound Care* 7(2): 81–4

Moffatt CJ, Franks PJ, Doherty DC, *et al* (2003) Lymphoedema: an underestimated health problem. *Q J Med* 96: 731–8

Moffat FL, Ketcham AS (1994) Surgery for malignant neoplasia: the evolution of oncologic surgery and its role in the management of cancer patients. In: Mc Kenna RJ, Murphey GP, eds. *Cancer Surgery*. PA Lippincott, Philadelphia: 1–20

Montrose PA (1987) Extravasation management. *Sem Oncol Nurs* 3(2): 128–32

Morison MJ, Moffatt CJ, Franks PJ (2007) *Leg Ulcers: a Problem-Based Learning Approach*. Mosby, Edinburgh

Naylor W, Laverty D, Mallett J (2001) *The Royal Marsden Hospital Handbook of Wound Management in Cancer Care*. Blackwell Science, Oxford

Neal K (1991) Treating fungating lesions. *Nurs Times* 87: 84–5

Olde Damink SWM, Soeters PB (1997) Nutrition and wound healing. *Nurs Times* 93(30): 1–6

Ottery FD (1995) Supportive nutrition to prevent cachexia and improve quality of life. *Sem Oncol* 3: 98–111

Otto S (2001) *Oncology Nursing*. 4th edn. Mosby, Philadelphia

Ovenson L, Hannibal J, Mortensen EL (1993) The inter-relationship of weight loss, dietary intake and quality of life in ambulatory patients with cancer of the lung, breast and ovary. *Nutr Cancer* 19: 159–67

Regnard C, Tempest S (1992) *A Guide to Symptom Relief in Advanced Cancer*. 3rd edn. Haigh and Hockland, London

Richardson A, Ream E, Wilson–Barnett J (1998) Fatigue in patients receiving chemotherapy: patterns of change. *Cancer Nurs* 21: 17–30

Seaman S (2006) Management of malignant fungating wounds in advanced cancer. *Sem Oncol Nurs* 22: 185–93

Senter H, Pringle A (1985) *How Wounds Heal: a Practical Guide for Nurses*. Wellcome Foundation, Cheshire

Sitton E (1992) Early and late radiation-induced skin alterations, part 1: mechanisms of skin changes. *Oncol Nurs Forum* 19(5): 801–7

Stoios N (1999) Prevention of extravasation in intravenous therapy: a review of the research evidence. In: Brighton D, Wood M (2005) *The Royal Marsden Hospital Handbook of Cancer Chemotherapy*. Churchill Livingstone, London

Stroemgren AS, Goldschmidt D, Groenvold M (2002) Self-assessment in cancer patients referred to palliative care: a study of feasibility and symptom epidemiology. *Cancer* **94**: 512–20

Thomas S (1997) A structured approach to the selection of dressings. World Wide Wounds. In: Naylor W, Laverty D, Mallett J (2001) *The Royal Marsden Hospital Handbook of Wound Management in Cancer Care*. Blackwell Science, Oxford

Veitch J (1993) Skin problems in lymphoedema. *Wound Management* **4**: 42–5

Winningham ML, Nail LM, Burke MB (1994) Fatigue and the cancer experience: the state of the knowledge. *Oncol Nurs Forum* **21**(1): 23–36

CHAPTER 10

HOLISTIC MANAGEMENT OF CHRONIC WOUND PAIN

Claire Acton

The pain experienced by a patient with a chronic wound can vary in nature and can have many causes (Hollinworth, 2005). The pain may be associated with traumatic wound procedures, for example, during wound debridement or dressing changes. This is usually short-lived (acute) and is a result of tissue damage. Such pain has been described as non-cyclic, if the procedure causing the pain is a single or an infrequent traumatic procedure, or cyclic if it is a regular occurrence (Krasner, 1995). Wound pain may also be persistent (chronic) and not associated with tissue trauma, for example, as a result of ongoing pathology, wound infection or chronic inflammation. Cyclic or non-cyclic pain is typically nociceptive in nature, with the pain diminishing and disappearing once the procedure causing the trauma has stopped. Persistent pain may also be nociceptive in nature due to continual stimulation of nociceptors in areas of ongoing tissue damage (Ashburn and Staats, 1999), but it can also persist long after the tissue damage that initially triggered its onset has resolved. This type of pain, which is a result of damage or dysfunction of nervous tissue, is called neuropathic pain.

Patient-focused care

Pain is the symptom that patients with chronic wounds find most distressing. Dressing changes are the most frequently cited cause (Price, 2005). However, there are many other individual factors to consider and dressing changes must be placed within the context of total pain management. The patient, and not just the wound, should be the focal point of care (Price, 2005; Price *et al*, 2007).

In the past, little attention has been given to the psychological and social needs of patients when carrying out wound care (Hollinworth and Hawkins, 2002). Emphasis has generally been on wound assessment and choice of dressing, rather than the assessment of the patient as a whole, for example their attitudes to the wound, the inconveniences it causes them, and the disruption it has on their everyday lives because of the pain and discomfort it causes (Benbow, 2006). Providing psychological support to help patients cope with the wound-related pain and emotional problems that may result is an important component of caring for the patient as a whole. Unfortunately, it is an area that has received little attention in clinical research (Hollinworth and Hawkins, 2002; Benbow, 2006).

Psychological aspects of pain

Because chronic pain is unrelenting, it is likely that stress, environmental and affective factors may be superimposed on the pain that arises from the original damaged tissue and contribute to its persistence and intensity (Loeser and Melzack, 1999). Persistent pain can profoundly affect a patient's mood, personality and social relationships (Ashburn and Staats, 1999). People with persistent pain typically experience concomitant depression, sleep disturbance, fatigue, and decreased overall physical functioning. Patients who are threatened by pain may suffer fear, anxiety and worry. Indeed, stress has been linked with delays in wound healing (Vileikyte, 2007). This is thought to be due to the disruption of the neuroendocrine immune equilibrium (Vileikyte, 2007) or, to a susceptibility to bacterial wound infection (Rojas *et al*, 2002). Those with marked fears of pain may avoid the behaviour which causes the pain, eg. avoiding movement or procedures that trigger the pain, which may increase disability and make matters worse. These patients may also exhibit anger, frustration, feelings of hopelessness and helplessness. These sequellae of pain have been discussed in detail (Australian and New Zealand College of Anaesthetists [ANZCA], 2005; Royal College of Surgeons, 2000).

Relieving pain with analgesics, for example, is only one of the many issues that must be addressed in the management of a patient with persistent pain. Patients may be helped by providing them with information which can help them to understand their pain, and by encouraging them to take an active role in its management (Eccleston, 2001). The goal of therapy is to control pain and to rehabilitate the patient so that they can function as well as possible (Ashburn and Staats, 1999). All the dimensions of the patient's condition should be treated. Behavioural and psychological therapies, such as cognitive behavioural therapy (CBT) should be integrated, wherever appropriate, into an interdisciplinary approach to treatment. Patients with chronic pain may require referral to a pain team if it is recalcitrant or difficult to control (Grey *et al*, 2006). However, its management should be considered the responsibility of all healthcare professionals involved with the patient, such as doctors, nurses, psychologists, physical and occupational therapists, vocational counsellors and pharmacists.

Pain assessment

Many factors influence a patient's sensation of pain, and it is difficult to objectively assess pain levels. Healthcare professionals need to take the time to engage and listen to patients. Understanding the patient's pain experience, and the effects it has on their daily lives is essential for identifying the most appropriate means for managing their pain and providing supportive measures. Because many patients find it difficult to describe their pain, giving them descriptive words to choose from and using a pain-measuring tool can help, and, if used on a regular basis, will enable the patient's progress to be monitored, thereby assessing the effectiveness of interventions. Changes in the level of pain may indicate a need to reassess the choice and timing of analgesics and/or other interventions used for managing the pain (World Union of Wound Healing Societies [WUWHS], 2004). All assessments made should be well documented to ensure effective communication between healthcare professionals and to maintain continuity of care for the patient which, in itself, will enhance the outcomes.

No single pain measuring scale is suitable for all patients; the choice will depend on the individual patient's needs and circumstances. However, once chosen, the same scale should be used for subsequent assessments (WUWHS, 2004).

The following are suggested key elements of pain assessment (Doughty, 2006):

* when and for how long the pain is experienced: this will identify particular procedures that cause or exacerbate the pain, and whether or not the pain is acute or persistent

- type of pain: to identify whether the pain is nociceptive or neuropathic or mixed in nature
- severity: establish the severity using an established rating scale, such as the numeric pain intensity scale, the visual analogue scale, or the faces rating scale (*Chapter 11*)
- the impact of pain on the patient: to identify the consequences of pain for their daily lives (eg. sleep, walking and work)
- factors which increase or decrease pain: these can give important clues to the wound aetiology (eg. to differentiate between venous and ischaemic ulcers)
- relief rating: assessment of scores after receiving analgesia can give a useful measure of interventions for pain management
- related adverse effects: to identify treatment-related adverse side-effects to enable appropriate measures to be taken to reduce their impact, such as giving alternative treatments, or treatments to alleviate the side-effects.

Price *et al* (2007) identify six critical dimensions for the assessment of pain: location, duration, intensity, quality, onset, and impact on activities of daily living. They also state that 'holistic management must be based on a safe and effective mix of psychosocial approaches together with local and systemic management'.

Unfortunately, the value of using a valid pain assessment tool appears to be unrecognised by many healthcare professionals. Results from an international survey, exploring wound care practitioners' understanding of pain and trauma at dressing changes, found that pain assessment was considered a low priority, with greater reliance being put on body language and non-verbal cues (Moffatt *et al*, 2002).

Treatment of pain

Pain in wounds can be caused, or is influenced by, many factors. These include disease processes, treatments and wound care procedure, types of wound management products used, emotional and social issues, and professional issues (Hollinworth, 2005). Treating all aspects of pain may not be possible, but it is important that as many factors as possible are considered and addressed. The fundamentals of pain management in wound care have been reviewed (Coulling, 2007).

Clearly, treating the underlying pathology causing the wound is desirable and is an effective strategy for removing pain resulting from chronic wounds. However, in many cases the prospect of eradicating the underlying cause of the wound (eg. venous insufficiency in leg ulcers or malignancy in fungating lesions) may be difficult, if not impossible. Therefore, other means of alleviating wound pain are required to relieve the pain symptoms. Infected wounds can be the source of inflammation and pain and eliminating the infection by use of appropriate antibiotics should help with this.

A regimen for relieving pain and associated stress should be developed for each individual patient, and may include several elements. Analgesics and/or psychological and other non-drug therapies can be considered on a continual or intermittent basis for relieving persistent or procedural pain respectively. As pain is particularly associated with dressing changes, care should be taken to adopt regimens for removal and replacement of dressings and cleaning/debriding the wound that minimise trauma to the wound. Ideally, the dressings in contact with the wound and surrounding skin should be easy to remove without causing additional damage to the wound and the sensitive surrounding skin. Interventions to reduce stress and emotional problems that are frequently associated with pain should also be considered, whether by drug treatment, such as anxiolytics and antidepressants or psychosocial therapy such as counselling or CBT.

For extremely painful procedures, such as the debridement of deep ulcers, it may be necessary to consider general anaesthesia, local neural blockade, spinal analgesia, or the use of mixed nitrous oxide and oxygen (Entonox).

Analgesics and anti-inflammatory drugs

Analgesics are the most common intervention for relieving pain, and can be given systemically on a continual basis for persistent wound pain. However, adverse effects, particularly with opioids, can be problematic. Systemic or topical analgesics or local anaesthetics can also be considered for reducing procedural pain. Because of the inflammatory nature of many chronic wounds, use of non-steroidal anti-inflammatory drugs (NSAIDS), such as ibuprofen, can also be considered with or without other analgesics (Popescu and Salcido, 2004). It should be remembered that if systemic drugs are used for treating procedural pain, sufficient doses should be used and sufficient time allowed for the drug to take effect.

In the absence of specific clinical trials in wound care, experience from treatment of chronic pain arising from other diseases can be used to guide choice for persistent wound pain. For pain that is nociceptive in nature, whether it arises from traumatic procedures or inflammation, analgesics should be considered and used promptly. Choice depends on the intensity of the pain. The World Health Organization has developed a three-step ladder for managing cancer pain and chronic pain, which it claims is effective in about 90% of patients (WHO, 2006). This uses drugs of increasing potency alone or in combination depending on severity, and titrated until the pain is controlled. Non-opioids (aspirin, paracetamol or NSAIDs) are used in the first instance for mild pain; then mild opioids, such as codeine, for moderate pain; and strong opioids, such as morphine, diamorphine, or fentanyl, for severe pain. Adjuvants are recommended in addition. These are not themselves analgesics, but they enhance the effect of analgesics by treating side-effects of opioids (for example, anti-emetics or laxatives) or treating other symptoms associated with pain, such as anxiolytics. Recently, topical corticosterioids have been found to relieve pain when applied directly to chronic leg ulcers, suggesting that the suppression of inflammation plays a role in pain relief (Hofman *et al*, 2007). Whatever analgesic drug is chosen, it is important that they are given in the appropriate dose and on a regular basis to control chronic pain, in accordance with their licensed doses and monitored accordingly. Details can be found in their summaries of product characteristics, which can be accessed online at www.medicines.org.uk.

Consultation with a pain specialist is advisable when opioids are required, in order to identify the optimum dose and form to use. The objective is to provide the necessary level and duration of pain relief, while minimising unacceptable side-effects. A recent meta-analysis of opioids for non-cancer pain found them to be effective in relieving pain associated with a wide range of diseases, and for both nociceptive and neuropathic pain. However, they were associated with many adverse effects. Constipation, nausea, dizziness or vertigo, somnolence and drowsiness, vomiting, dry skin, itching or pruritus, and sedation all occurred more frequently with opioids than with placebo (Furlan *et al*, 2006).

Neuropathic pain is often difficult to relieve, not just because of its severity, but because it is generally resistant to simple analgesics. Although opioids may help, alternative non-analgesic treatments can be tried. These include local anaesthetics, gabapentin, pregabalin, tricyclic antidepressants, such as amitriptyline, and mixed serotonin-noradrenaline reuptake inhibitors, such as venlafaxine (Gilron *et al*, 2006). A Cochrane review considered that carbamazepine, an anticonvulsant medicine, was effective for relieving pain caused by damage to nerves, either from injury or disease. However, the trials supporting its use have been small (Wiffen *et al*, 2005).

Opioid receptors are present in peripheral nerves, and become susceptible to the action of opioids during inflammation. In chronic wounds, where inflammation is generally present, topical opioids offer a means to relieve localised wound pain while minimising the risk of systemic side-effects (Ashfield, 2005). A number of cases of the successful use of topical opioids have been reported, although there have been no well-controlled randomised studies. For example, Twillman *et al* (Twillman *et al*, 1999) reported immediate pain relief in seven out of nine patients with painful skin ulcers when 0.1% morphine-infused gel was applied. There are several other reports of the successful use of morphine or diamorphine topical gels (Flock, 2003; Abbas, 2004; Ashfield, 2005), however, the number of people in these studies is small. Gallagher *et al* (2005) reported the use of methadone mixed with Stomahesive powder (ConvaTec). Sprinkling this mixture onto open wounds at the time of dressing changes was claimed to be effective for 24 hours or more, without adverse side-effects. It should be remembered that opioids are not currently licensed for topical use in this way, and there is no good evidence to guide choice of dosage or any particular mode of delivery.

Topical anaesthetics may be suitable for use before painful intermittent procedures. Use of eutectic mixture of lidocaine and prilocaine (EMLA) (Astra Zeneca) has been evaluated for the relief of pain occurring during debridement of venous leg ulcers in a number of studies. A Cochrane review concluded that EMLA did provide effective pain relief for venous leg ulcer debridement, but the effect of the product on ulcer healing was unknown (Briggs and Nelson, 2003). Again, the use of such anaesthetics topically in wound management is not licensed. No trials that address the treatment of persistent pain (between and at dressing changes) were identified.

Growing evidence for the effectiveness of a foam dressing containing ibuprofen to reduce pain (Biatain-Ibu [Coloplast]) is available from two small studies. In a prospective case series study, 10 patients with painful chronic venous leg ulcers were treated for six dressing changes with Biatain-Ibu. The ibuprofen dressing demonstrated a reduction in pain intensity scores during the study, but this increased one week after discontinuing treatment (Flanagan *et al*, 2006). In another study — a small single-blinded crossover study of 12 patients — use of the ibuprofen dressing was reported to be associated with a statistically significant decrease in pain intensity compared with a placebo. In a multinational double blind study involving 122 patients, a foam dressing impregnated with ibuprofen was found to be successful in providing persistent pain relief (Gottrup *et al*, 2007). Although having the advantage of convenience, the use of a proprietary dressing containing ibuprofen has limitations. It does not allow for dose modification of the NSAID or the use of other, and possibly more appropriate, dressing types depending on the wound characteristics. As with other topical pain-relieving strategies, more extensively and appropriately powered studies are required to establish its side-effect profile and identify its role in management of wound pain (Jørgensen *et al*, 2006).

Psychological and other non-drug therapies

Psychological factors are important modifiers of pain perception, and thus psychological therapies can complement other pain-relieving measures (Adams *et al*, 2006). These therapies focus upon emotional, cognitive and behavioural aspects of illness, addressing beliefs through education about their condition, reducing anxiety and stress by teaching stress management techniques, and improving personal control by teaching coping skills (Adams *et al*, 2006). There are a wide range of psychological approaches that can be considered, and these include psychophysiological, behavioural, cognitive behavioural and psychodynamic therapies.

Cognitive behavioural therapy is well recognised as an intervention that can be helpful for a wide range of psychological problems, and is probably the most widely used therapy in pain management programmes. CBT attempts to change the negative thoughts and dysfunctional attitudes to foster more healthy and adaptive thoughts, emotions and actions in the patients (Ashburn and Staats, 1999). A systemic review and meta-analysis of 25 studies, including 1672 patients with chronic pain (excluding headache) found significant benefits of CBT over both waiting list controls and alternative treatments with regard to measures of pain and several other (but not all) quality of life domains. Interpretation of the results is uncertain, because of the variations of study design and comparator treatments used in the included studies (Morley *et al*, 1999). Any CBT undertaken requires the patient to be an active participant in the process rather than a passive recipient so may not be suitable for all patients.

Relaxation techniques are a common component of multimodal chronic pain management, and have been suggested, among other interventions, as an option for managing wound pain (Krasner, 1995). However, there appears to be no good evidence for its effectiveness. A systematic review of randomised, controlled trials, including patients with malignant and non-malignant pain, failed to identify any significant benefits compared with other interventions for relieving chronic pain (Carroll and Seers, 1998).

Frenay *et al* (2001) compared hypnosis with stress-reducing strategies administered by a psychologist to alleviate pain during dressing changes of patients with 10–25% body surface area burns, as adjunctive treatments to analgesics and anxiolytics. Hypnosis was found to be more effective than the stress-reducing strategies at reducing anxiety before and during dressing changes. Although both treatments were considered to improve pain and patient satisfaction, there was no difference between them in these respects.

Transcutaneous electrical nerve stimulation (TENS) is widely used in the treatment of many types of chronic pain, sometimes as a first-line treatment. However, a Cochrane review of 19 studies that met suitable quality inclusion criteria found insufficient evidence to draw any conclusions about its analgesic effectiveness for the treatment of chronic pain in adults. The reviewers considered that new trials of better design are needed before any evidence-based recommendations can be made for patients or healthcare professionals for the treatment of chronic pain (Carroll *et al*, 2000).

There are many other alternative or complementary therapies that may have a role in the holistic management of chronic wounds. These include acupuncture, energy healing, physical therapy, distraction (eg. using music), guided imagery, biofeedback, and mediation or prayer (Krasner 1995; Papantonio, 1998). There appears to be no robust clinical trial evidence to support the use of any of these therapies for relieving pain in wound care.

Wound care procedures

Dressing removal and wound cleansing are the most painful wound care interventions (Hollinworth and Collier, 2000; Kammerlander and Eberlein, 2002; Moffatt *et al*, 2002). Furthermore, anticipation of a painful wound care procedure can lead to considerable apprehension and stress. Talking to patients about pain and how much they can expect, together with an explanation of whatever measures are in place to minimise pain will help reduce fear and anxiety (Briggs *et al*, 2002).

There are a number of simple measures that can be used for reducing anxiety during painful procedures (Smith *et al*, 1997):

- identify what the patient recognises as triggers of pain and pain reducers
- invite patient involvement to the extent desired by the patient
- encourage slow, rhythmic breathing during the procedure
- allow the patient to pace the procedure, offering 'time-outs' that are requested through verbal or non-verbal communication.

The opinion of an expert working group of the WUWHS was published as a consensus document Minimising Pain at Wound Dressing-Related Procedures in 2004 (WUWHS, 2004). This document points out that preparation and planning of the dressing change procedures are key to effective pain management, and suggests the following measures:

- choose an appropriate non-stressful environment. Close windows, turn off mobile phones, etc
- explain to the patient in simple terms what will be done and the method that will be used
- assess the need for skilled or unskilled assistance, such as someone to simply hold the patient's hand
- be thoughtful in positioning the patient to minimise discomfort and avoid unnecessary contact or exposure
- avoid prolonged exposure of the wound, eg. waiting for specialist advice
- avoid any unnecessary stimulus to the wound. Handle wounds gently, being aware that any slight touch can cause pain
- involve the patient throughout. Frequent verbal checks and use of pain tools offer real-time feedback
- consider preventive analgesia.

In view of the pain and trauma that results from changing wound dressings, it is important to restrict dressing changes to those that are necessary. The desire to see what the wound looks like has to be balanced against the damage that may be caused to the wound and the surrounding skin by removing the dressing, and the pain and stress inflicted on the patient by the change procedure. Using an adhesive remover spray or wipe will significantly reduce pain of this type. It is used widely in stoma care and is becoming more popular in wound care. Use of non-adherent primary contact layers, which can be left in place at dressing changes, and require only the secondary absorbent layer to be removed, offers a useful means of reducing wound trauma. Mepitel® (Mölnlycke) is an atraumatic soft-silicone non-adherent wound contact dressing, which can be left in place for up to 14 days (Platt *et al*, 1996; Bugmann *et al*, 1998; Terrill and Varughese, 2000). It allows exudate to pass through it, while maintaining a moist wound environment. Although Mepitel does not adhere to the wound bed, it does adhere to adjacent dry healthy skin (Pudner, 2001). When wet, Mepitel becomes transparent and allows wound healing to be monitored with minimal trauma at intermediate dressing changes.

Much of the pain and trauma occurring during dressing changes may be obviated by appropriate selection of dressings that allow moist wound healing and do not use aggressive adhesives (see next section); this avoids the often unsuccessful approach of soaking dressing in water or saline to effect removal (Hollinworth, 2005).

Pain to the wound and periwound skin during dressing changes can also occur as a result of applying wound irrigation and cleansing solutions. Use of irritant or allergic materials should be avoided where possible (Conway and Whettam, 2002). Although use of sterile normal saline is an appropriate cleansing solution, a review found that wound cleansing with water was no different from cleansing with normal saline, any other solution, or indeed no cleansing, with regard to rates of healing and infection (Fernandez *et al*, 2002). If tap water is used for wound cleansing, then the quality must be considered (Betts, 2003). The temperature of the solution should be warm, not only for comfort but to prevent the arrest of the healing process which can happen for some hours after a dressing change (McKirdy, 2001).

Choice of dressings

By careful selection of dressings much of the pain and trauma associated with wound dressing changes can be avoided. An international survey of wound care practitioners identified the following (Moffatt *et al*, 2002):

- dried out dressings and adherent products were the most likely to cause pain and trauma at dressing changes
- pain-free removal was considered the most desirable characteristic of a dressing

- there appeared to be a close association between those dressings that caused wound trauma and those that caused pain
- gauze was the most likely to cause both pain and trauma and hydrogels, hydrofibres and alginates and soft silicones were the least likely
- use of atraumatic dressings was considered the most important strategy to avoid wound damage
- the most common strategy to manage pain was to soak old dressings, just ahead of selecting non-traumatic dressings and choosing dressings that offered pain-free removal.

Many of these findings may reflect the continued use of gauze as a wound dressing in many centres, despite the current recommended practice of using dressings that promote moist wound healing.

Removal of dressings that have adhered to the wound destroys newly-formed granulation tissue and newly-formed fragile capillary loops that have penetrated the dressing material (Collier and Hollinworth, 2000). Although use of gauze is particularly problematic, patients continue to experience pain and trauma with the use of some of the modern wound dressings, many of which can adhere to the wound if they dry out. It is necessary to choose a secondary dressing carefully when required, as this could have an effect on the moisture level maintenance at the wound bed and the overall performance of the primary dressing.

Adverse irritant or allergic reactions to wound dressings or auxiliary wound care products can occur. If the skin reaction is a result of an allergic rather than an irritant reaction, it may only be seen after a few days or on repeated application. Identification of the agent causing the irritation/sensitisation reaction is desirable, so that wound care products can be chosen that do not contain this material (Conway and Whettam, 2002). Skin barrier function is compromised in skin that is subject to excoriation and stripping, as a result of repeated application and removal of adhesive products which increases the likelihood of adverse skin reactions. Different dressings vary considerably with regard to their skin-stripping potential and the level of discomfort experienced on removal. It should be considered standard practice to apply a skin barrier product to prevent this and to help extend the dressing wear time. However, at least on normal skin, these two properties appear to be poorly correlated. For example, Mepilex border (Mölnlycke) (a soft silicone adhesive product) produced less discomfort on removal than DuoDERM® Extra Thin (ConvaTec),

Biatain® (Coloplast) and Versiva® (ConvaTec), although peel forces were similar (Dykes and Heggie, 2003).

It is important that dressings are chosen that promote moist wound healing (WUWHS, 2004). By choosing a dressing that maintains a moist wound healing environment, and that does not dry out, the friction at the wound surface will be reduced and this will minimise wound trauma and pain on removal (Briggs *et al*, 2002). Choice of a dressing that can stay *in situ* for a longer period to avoid frequent removal may also be appropriate (Briggs *et al*, 2002). It is, of course, important that the dressings are changed before they become saturated, leak and allow spread of potentially corrosive exudate onto the periwound skin. If a skin barrier product was used this would not be an issue. Should soaking be required, or there is bleeding or trauma to the wound or surrounding skin, or pain is a problem on removal, the choice of dressing should be reconsidered (Briggs *et al*, 2002; WUWHS, 2004).

Fibrous products (alginates and hydrofibres) form a gel in contact with wound exudate, and are excellent non-adherent contact layers, and generally provide good pain relief (Reddy *et al*, 2003). However, they can also become strongly adherent and cause wound trauma on removal should they dry out, for example, if the exudate level reduces. Hydrogel sheets and other non-adherent layers can also be used effectively for reducing adhesion to the wound and preventing damage and pain on removal.

Preventing trauma on removal from wounds and surrounding skin has led many manufacturers to modify their adhesive to reduce trauma on removal (Hollinworth, 2006). Soft silicone dressings were developed specifically with this in mind, and have low peel strengths to reduce damage to delicate periwound skin. Such dressings are now appropriately designated as 'atraumatic' dressings, and they are the first-choice dressing for preventing wound trauma. Mepitel was the first of the atraumatic dressings to be introduced. It consists of a flexible polyamide net coated with soft silicone. Mepitel has been shown to cause significantly less pain on removal from skin grafts, burns, surgical wounds, and traumatic wounds (Dahlstrøm, 1995; Williams, 1995; Platt *et al*, 1996; Gotschall *et al*, 1998). This product also has been used successfully in the management of extensive mycosis fungoides (cutaneous T-cell lymphoma) of the face and scalp (Taylor, 1999). Further extensive evidence to support the use of soft-silicone dressings can be found in the reviews by Thomas (2003) and White (2005), and its safe use in a wide variety of wounds is reflected in a current clinical best practice statement (Independent Advisory Group, 2004).

Conclusion and summary

Pain is a frequent cause of psychological distress in patients with chronic wounds and can severely affect quality of life. Minimising trauma and pain should be a key objective of healthcare professionals involved in the care of patients with chronic wounds, and a major factor in relieving psychological distress, at, between, or in anticipation of wound dressing changes. Evidence to support the use of therapies (analgesics or psychological therapies) to relieve pain in chronic wounds is limited and mostly comes from extrapolation of results from studies of the treatment of chronic pain in other diseases, and from expert opinion. It is recommended that a holistic approach should be taken to pain management.

It is important to understand the causes of the pain and provide, where appropriate, interventions to minimise pain, before, during and after wound care procedures. Analgesics should be chosen to relieve acute and persistent pain and adjunctive use of psychological and other non-drug therapies considered. As dressing changes are the most frequent cause of pain in wound management, particular attention should be given to the selection of a dressing and dressing change regimen that reduce the likelihood of trauma to the wound and the skin surrounding it. Dressings that provide moist wound healing should be chosen. Soft silicone dressings are recognised as the dressings least likely to cause trauma to the wound and surrounding skin, and should be considered as the first choice for the treatment of painful chronic wounds.

References

Abbas SQ (2004) Diamorphine-Intrasite dressings for painful pressure ulcers. *J Pain Symptom Manage* 28: 532–4

Adams N, Poole H, Richardson C (2006) Psychological approaches to chronic pain management: part 1. *J Clin Nurs* 15(3): 290–300

Australian and New Zealand College of Anaesthetists (2005) *Acute pain maangement: scientific evidence*. Department of Health, Australia. Available online at: www.anzca.edu.au/publications/acutepain.pdf (last accessed 22 October 2007)

Ashburn MA, Staats PS (1999) Management of chronic pain. *Lancet* 353: 1865–9

Ashfield T (2005) The use of topical opioids to relieve pressure ulcer pain. *Nurs Standard* 19: 90–2

Benbow M (2006) Holistic assessment of pain and chronic wounds. *J Comm Nurs* **20**: 24–8

Betts J (2003) Review: wound cleansing with water does not differ from no cleansing or cleansing with other solutions for rates of wound infection or healing. *Evidence-based Nurs* **6**(3): 81

Briggs M, Nelson EA (2003) *Topical agents or dressings for pain in venous leg ulcers.* Cochrane Database Syst Rev 1: CD001177. DOI: 10.1002/14651858.CD001177

Briggs M, Torra i Bou JE (2002) Pain at wound dressing changes: a guide to management. In: *Pain at Wound Dressing Changes.* European Wound Management Association Position Document. MEP Ltd, London

Bugmann PH, Taylor S, Gyger D, *et al* (1998) A silicone-coated nylon dressing reduces healing time in burned paediatric patients. *Burns* **24**: 609–12

Carroll D, Moore RA, McQuay HJ, *et al* (2000) *Transcutaneous electrical nerve stimulation (TENS) for chronic pain.* Cochrane Database Syst Rev 4: CD003222. DOI: 10.1002/14651858.CD003222

Carroll D, Seers K (1998) Relaxation for the relief of chronic pain: a systematic review. *J Adv Nurs* **87**: 476–87

Collier M, Hollinworth H (2000) Pain and tissue trauma during dressing changes. *Nurs Standard* **14**: 71–3

Coulling S (2007) Fundamentals of pain management in wounds. *Br J Nurs* (Tissue Viability Supplement) **16**(11): S4–S12

Conway J, Whettam J (2002) Adverse reactions to wound dressings. *Nurs Standard* **16**: 52–60

Dahlstrøm KK (1995) A new silicone rubber dressing used as a temporary dressing before delayed split skin grafting. A prospective randomised study. *Scand J Plast Reconstr Surg Hand Surg* **29**: 325–7

Doughty DB (2006) Strategies for minimizing chronic wound pain. *Adv Skin Wound Care* **19**: 82–5

Dykes PJ, Heggie R (2003) The link between the peel force of adhesive dressings and subjective discomfort in volunteer subjects. *J Wound Care* **12**: 260–2

Eccleston C (2001) Role of psychology in pain management. *Br J Anaesth* **87**: 144–52

Fernandez R, Griffiths R, Ussia C (2002) *Water for wound cleansing.* Cochrane Database Syst Rev 4: CD003861 DOI: 10.1002/14651858. CD003861

Flanagan M, Vogensen H, Haase L, *et al* (2006) *Case series investigating the experience of pain in patients with chronic venous leg ulcers treated with a foam dressing releasing ibuprofen.* World Wide Wounds. Available online at: www.worldwidewounds.com/2006/april/Flanagan/Ibuprofen-Foam-Dressing.html (last accessed 23 November 2006)

Flock P (2003) Pilot study to determine the effectiveness of diamorphine gel to control pressure ulcer pain. *J Pain Symptom Manage* 25: 547–54

Frenay MC, Faymonville ME, Devlieger S, Albert A, Vanderkelen A (2001) Psychological approaches during dressing changes: a prospective randomised study comparing hypnosis against stress-reducing strategies. *Burns* 27(8): 793–9

Furlan AD, Sandoval JA, Mailis-Gagnon A, Tunks E (2006) Opioids for chronic noncancer pain: a meta-analysis of effectiveness and side effects. *CMAJ* 174: 189–94

Gallagher RE, Arndt DR, Hunt KL (2005) Analgesic effects of topical methadone. A report of four cases. *Clin J Pain* 21: 190–2

Gilron I, Watson PN, Cahill CM, Moulin DE (2006) Neuropathic pain: a practical guide for the clinician. *CMAJ* 175(3): 265–75

Gotschall CS, Morrison MIS, Eichelberger MR (1998) Prospective randomized study of the efficacy of Mepitel and children with partial-thickness scalds. *J Burn Care Rehabil* 19: 279–83

Gottrupp F, Jorgenson , Karlsmark T, et al (2007) Less pain with Biatain-Ibu: initial findings from a randomized controlled double blind clinical investigation on painful venous leg ulcers. *Int Wound J* 4(suppl 1): 24–34

Grey JE, Enoch S, Harding KG (2006) Wound assessment. *Br Med J* 332(7536): 285–8

Hofman D, Moore K, Cooper R, Eagle M, Cooper S (2007) Use of topical corticosteroids on chronic leg ulcers. *J Wound Care* 16(5): 227–30

Hollinworth H, Collier M (2000) Nurses' views about pain and trauma at dressing changes: results of a national survey. *J Wound Care* 9: 369–73

Hollinworth H, Hawkins J (2002) Teaching nurses psychological support of patients with wounds. *Br J Nurs* 11(suppl): S8–18

Hollinworth H (2006) Addressing pain and tissue trauma during wound care. *Nurs Resident Care* 8: 259–64

Hollinworth H (2005) The management of patients' pain in wound care. *Nurs Standard* 20: 65–73

Independent Advisory Group (2004) *Best Practice Statement: Minimising Trauma and Pain in Wound Management*. Wounds UK Ltd, Aberdeen

Jørgensen B, Friis GJ, Gottrup F (2006) Pain and quality of life for patients with venous leg ulcers: proof of concept of the efficacy of Biatain-Ibu, a new pain reducing wound dressing. *Wound Rep Regen* 14: 233–9

Kammerlander G, Eberlein T (2002) Nurses' views about pain at dressing changes: a central European perspective. *J Wound Care* 11: 76–9

Krasner D (1995) The chronic wound pain experience. *Ostomy/Wound Management* **41**: 20–5

Loeser JD, Melzack R (1999) Pain: an overview. *Lancet* **353**: 1607–9

McKirdy L (2001) Wound Mangement; burn wound cleansing. *J Community Nurs* **15**(5): 24–9

Moffatt CJ, Franks, Hollinworth H (2002) Understanding wound pain and trauma: an international perspective. In: *Pain At Wound Dressing Changes*. European Wound Management Association Position Document. MEP Ltd, London

Morley S, Eccleston C, Williams A (1999) Systematic review and meta-analysis of randomized controlled trials of cognitive behavioural therapy and behaviour therapy for chronic pain in adults. *Pain* **80**: 1–13

Papantonio C (1998) Alternative medicine and wound healing. *Ostomy/ Wound Management* **44**: 44–55

Platt AJ, Phipps A, Judkins K (1996) A comparative study of silicone net dressings and paraffin gauze dressing in skin-grafted sites. *Burns* **22**: 543–5

Popescu AP, Salcido R (2004) Wound pain: a challenge for the patient and the wound care specialist. *Adv Skin Wound Care* **17**: 14–20

Price P (2005) An holistic approach to wound pain in patients with chronic wounds. *Wounds* **17**: 55–7

Price P, Fogh K, Glynn B, *et al* (2007) Managing painful leg wounds: the Wound Pain Management Model. *Int Wound J* **4**(suppl 1): 4–15

Pudner R (2001) Low/non-adherent dressings in wound management. *J Community Nurs Online* **15**(8). Available online at: www.jcn.co.uk/j (last accessed 9 December 2006)

Reddy M, Kohr R, Queen D, Keast D, Sibbald RG (2003) Practical treatment of wound pain and trauma: a patient-centred approach. An overview. *Ostomy/Wound Management* **49**(4 Suppl): 2–15

Rojas IG, Padeett DA, Sheridan JF (2002) Stress-induced susceptibility to bacterial infection during wound healing. *Brain Behav Immun* **16**(1): 74–84

Royal College of Surgeons of England (2000) *Report on the working party pain after surgery*. Royal College of Surgeons of England, London. Available online at: www.rcseng.ac.uk/rcseng/content/publications/docs/ pain_after_surgery.html (last accessed 20 October 2007)

Smith NK, Pasero CL, McCaffery M (1997) Non-drug measures for painful procedures. *Am J Nurs* **97**: 18–20

Soon K, Acton C (2006) Pain-induced stress: a barrier to wound healing. *Wounds UK* **2**(4): 92–101

Taylor R (1999) Use of a silicone net dressing in severe mycosis fungoides. *J Wound Care* **8**: 429–30

Terrill PJ, Varughese G (2000) A comparison of three primary non-adherent dressings applied to hand surgery wounds. *J Wound Care* 9(8): 359–63

Thomas S (2003) *Atraumatic dressings*. World Wide Wounds. Available online at: www.worldwidewounds.com/2003/january/Thomas/Atraumatic-Dressings.html (last accessed 23 November 2006)

Twillman RK, Long TD, Cathers TA, Mueller DW (1999) Treatment of painful skin ulcers with topical opioids. *J Pain Symptom Manage* 17(4): 288–92

Vileikyte L (2007) Stress and wound healing. *Clin Dermatol* 25(1): 49–55

White R (2005) Evidence for atraumatic soft silicone wound dressing use. *Wounds UK* 1: 104–9

Wiffen PJ, McQuay HJ, Moore RA (2005) *Carbamazepine for acute and chronic pain*. Cochrane Database Syst Rev 3: CD005451. DOI: 10.1002/14651858.CD005451

Williams C (1995) Mepitel: a non-adherent soft silicone wound dressing. *Br J Nurs* 4(1): 51–5

World Union of Wound Healing Societies (2004) *Principles of Best Practice 2004: Minimising Pain at Wound Dressing-related Procedures*. A Consensus Document. MEP Ltd, London

World Health Organization (2006) *Palliative care*. WHO, Geneva. Available online at: www.who.int/cancer/palliative/en/ (last accessed 23 November 2006)

CHAPTER 11

PAINS-TAKING CARE: EVERYDAY ISSUES IN WOUND PAIN MANAGEMENT

Trudie Young and Andy Roden

Wound pain has a significant impact on the quality of life of individuals (Franks and Moffatt, 1998) and it has been established that clients with wounds such as leg ulcers experience significant greater bodily pain than the non-wounded population (Lindholm *et al*, 1993). Unfortunately, nurses may be unwilling to accept the degree of suffering caused by wound pain and consequently fail to manage it effectively. This chapter aims to guide the clinician through the assessment and management of wound pain. Pain is influenced by physiological, psychological, social and emotional factors.

Definition of pain

The International Association for the Study of Pain (IASP, 2006) describes pain as:

An unpleasant sensory and emotional experience associated with actual or potential tissue damage, or described in terms of such damage.

Physiology of wound pain

If we focus on wound pain there are two main types: nociceptive pain and neuropathic pain. However, these are not exclusive and a client may present with both elements to their pain. Stimuli from the periphery (mechanical, chemical, thermal) are transmitted to the spinal cord through the sensory afferent nerves. These afferents synapse on the dorsal horn second order neurons in the spinal column, which form pathways extending to the brain, primarily thalamus and somatosensory cortex.

Chronic pain is not just a prolonged acute pain, it is a distinct entity, with many functional and structural alterations of the peripheral and central nervous system. Central hyper-excitability is the key process in the generation of chronic pain. It is mediated in the second order dorsal horn neurons. *Figure 11.1* shows the pain pathways.

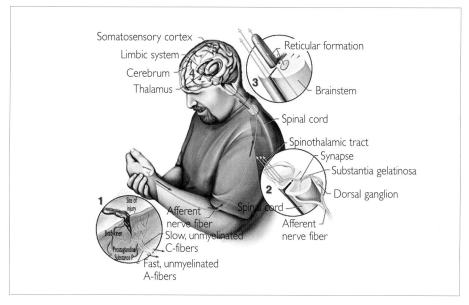

Figure 11.1: Pain pathways (Hamilton, 2006)

Pain sensations can be broadly divided up into bright, sharp, stabbing types of pain, and dull, throbbing, aching types. A-delta fibres mediate the former or 'fast' pain, for example, a pin-prick. C-fibres signal the latter or 'slow pain', such as the throbbing pain of a thumb hit with a hammer. However, not all A-delta and C-fibres are nociceptors. Some respond to low threshold stimuli such as touching or brushing, and repetitive and intense activation of the high-threshold C-fibres may cause the phenomenon of 'wind up' (which is an augmented response of the dorsal horn neurons to the same intensity stimuli). Reorganisation or remodelling of the synapses at the dorsal horn level, as well as at the brainstem, thalamus, and somatosensory cortex levels, is a well-documented phenomenon, referred to as 'neuronal plasticity', responsible for a variety of chronic pain syndromes (Fulgosi, 2006; Anaesthesia UK, 2006).

Plasticity may be described in terms of change in neuronal structure, or connections between the neurons. This, allied to changes in the neurotransmitters may result in increased activity of neurons, which in turn may result in increased pain. Injury, inflammation, and disease may all cause plasticity and therefore increase pain. McQuay and Dickinson (1990) proposed that pain is a memory and may be stored in the nervous system and that preventing such a memory being laid down may help pre-empting postoperative pain. McQuay and Dickinson (1990) also note that this may have implications when choosing the most appropriate method of providing analgesia, eg. if the pain memory is stored at a 'central' level, for instance in the brain, then attacking the pain in the leg or arm where it originated might not do any good.

Nociceptive pain

This is often referred to as acute pain that occurs following a painful event and is time limited. A typical example would be the pain experienced following removal of a dressing that had adhered to the wound bed. The pain would be incident related and disappear after a short period of time and the pain is eased by analgesia. *Figure 11.2* is a pain assessment algorithm and *Table 11.1* gives guidance on control regimes for nociceptive pain.

Neuropathic pain

This is an abnormal pain response in which the usual channels and processes for feeling, transmitting and interpreting pain have gone haywire. It is often found in people whose wounds have been open for some time. Neuropathic pain results in people having excruciating pain in their wound bed (hyperalgesia) or in the surrounding skin (allodynia). This severe pain can occur following what is normally perceived as a non-painful event, ie. exposure to the air for a few minutes. For these patients, conventional analgesia aimed at tissue-based pain may not ease the pain and they require different agents aimed at modifying nerve impulse transmission and often mixed agents, some of which are not traditional analgesics, eg. amitryptyline (see *Table 11.2* for neuropathic pain control regimes).

Table 11.1: Nociceptive pain control, regimes 1 and 2

Drug	Dose	Notes
Regime 1. Nociceptive, based on patient not currently taking any medication — use both medications in the regime simultaneously		
Paracetamol 1 g qds (two tablets 4–6-hourly)	Maximum eight in 24 hours	Do not exceed eight tablets Caution when taking other paracetamol containing products, eg. Kapake® (Galen) Caution in cases of chronic pancreatitis Liquid or soluble available
Plus		
Ibuprofen 400 mg TDS (one tablet every 8 hours)	Maximum three in 24 hours	Many trade names, eg. Motrin, Nurofen Caution in: renal disease, GI tract problems, heart failure May cause wheeze and tight chest in asthmatics — seek advice from pharmacist or doctor Take with food Syrup available
Regime 2. Nociceptive (based on patient having found regime 1 ineffective — use co-codamol at either strength with ibuprofen)		
Co-codamol 8/500 (8 mg codeine and 500 mg of paracetamol) (two tablets 4–6-hourly)	Maximum eight in 24 hours	'Over-the-counter medicine' — many trade names, for example, 'Paracodol®', 'Solpadeine', 'Panadeine®', etc Do not exceed eight tablets in 24 hours. Caution when taking other paracetamol containing products In cases of chronic pancreatitis, see pharmacist or doctor if previously had problems
If pain remains unchanged, change to: Co-codamol 30/500 (30 mg codeine and 500 mg paracetamol) (two tablets 4–6-hourly)	Maximum eight in 24 hours	Prescription-only medicine Also known as 'Kapake' 'Solpadol®' (Sanofi-Synthelabo) 'Tylex®' (Schwarz) Co-codamol 30/500 at eight tablets in 24 hours = 20–25 mg morphine per day equivalent If pain persists, see GP who may consider slow-release morphine preparations, eg. MST supplemented by regular paracetamol May cause constipation and nausea
Plus		
Ibuprofen 400 mg TDS (one tablet every 8 hours)	Maximum three in 24 hours	Many trade names, eg. 'Motrin' 'Nurofen' Caution in: renal disease, GI tract problems, heart failure May cause wheeze and tight chest in asthmatics — seek advice from pharmacist or doctor Take with food Syrup available

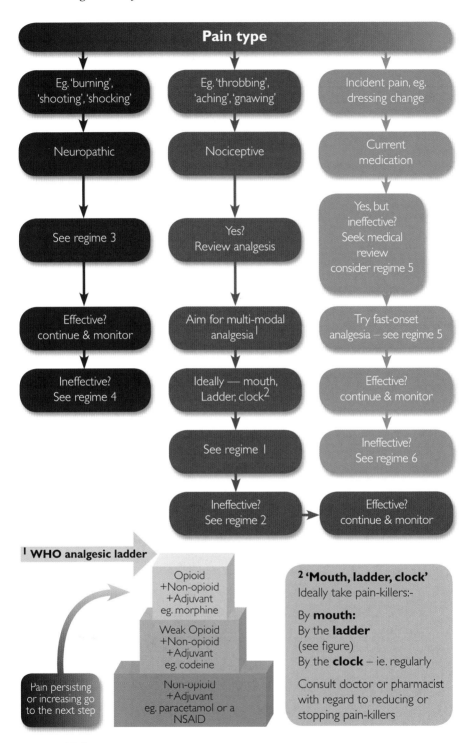

Figure 11.2: Pain assessment

Table 11.2: Neuropathic pain control, regimes 3 and 4

Drug	Dose	Notes
Regime 3. Neuropatic (+/- nociceptive), based on patient not currently taking medication — use all the medications simultaneously whether or not the patient has concurrent nociceptive pain		
Paracetamol 1g qds (two tablets 4–6-hourly)	Maximum eight in 24 hours	Do not exceed eight tablets Caution when taking other paracetamol containing products, eg. Kapake® (Galen) Caution in cases of chronic pancreatitis. Seek advice if unsure Liquid or soluble available
Plus		
Ibuprofen 400mg TDS (one tablet every 8 hours)	Maximum three in 24 hours	Many trade names, eg. Motrin, Nurofen Caution in: renal disease, GI tract problems, heart failure May cause wheeze and tight chest in asthmatics — seek advice from pharmacist or doctor Take with food Syrup available
Plus		
Amitryptyline 10mg at night (one tablet)	10–25mg	Antidepressant at high doses (at least double) May cause drowsiness, dry mouth, sedation in elderly Possibly may have no effect on 'nerve pain' until taken for two weeks. Avoid in arrhythmias or heart block Unlicensed use, but well-supported by evidence Start on 10mg increase after three weeks if ineffective
Regime 4. Neuropathic (+/- nociceptive), based on patient having found regime 3 ineffective, use all the medications simultaneously, regardless of the patient having nociceptive pain		
Paracetamol 1g QDS (two tablets 4–6-hourly)	Maximum eight in 24 hours	Do not exceed eight tablets Caution other paracetamol containing products, eg. 'Kapake' Caution in: chronic pancreatitis — seek advice if unsure Liquid or soluble available
Plus		
Ibuprofen 400mg TDS (one tablet every 8 hours)	Maximum three in 24 hours	Many trade names, eg. 'Motrin', 'Nurofen' Caution in: renal disease, GI tract problems, heart failure May cause wheeze and tight chest in asthmatics — seek advice from pharmacist or doctor Take with food. Syrup available
Plus		
Gabapentin (see dosing notes across*)	Up to 2.4g in 24 hours	Anti-convulsant. Licensed for neuropathic pain Good evidence Caution in: CCF, reduced dose in renal impairment Side-effects: dry mouth, sedation, nausea *Start 100mg at night for 3 nights; Then 100mg twice a day for 3 days; Then 100mg three times a day for 3 days, after which GP review effect vs side-effects to increase/decrease dose (ie. titrate dose to lessen side-effects)

Wound pain assessment

How can we differentiate between these different types of pain during our patient assessment? Before we look at this we must look at the overall assessment of a person in pain. The World Union of Wound Healing Societies (WUWHS) (2004) suggests we use a layered approach to pain assessment which involves an initial assessment, an ongoing assessment and a review assessment. The pain pyramid (*Figure 11.3*) provides a structure to help us understand the impact wound pain can have on the individual.

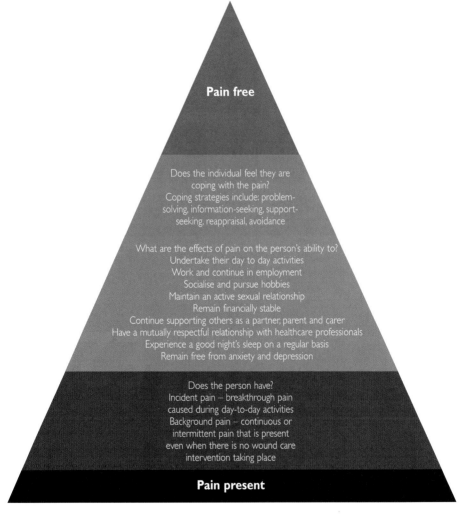

Figure 11.3: Pain pyramid

An individual's wound pain may be a one-off event or present throughout a 24-hour period. *Figure 11.4* highlights pain triggers (normal text) and reducers (bold text) that may be present around the clock.

Pain assessment tools

It is difficult to assess the impact of a person's pain on their life during a brief assessment period. However, we could ask the person to provide us with an insight into the wider implications of having wound pain. In addition, we can use pain assessment tools to help establish the severity of the pain, thus assessing its sensory dimension.

Pain assessment tools come in a number of main formats (*Table 11.3*):

- visual analogue scale
- numerical rating scales
- happy faces
- coloured ladder
- verbal rating scales.

In addition to the tools, we can use a set of descriptors to help the person describe their pain. These descriptors can also help to identify whether the pain is nociceptive or neuropathic, for example:

Nociceptive descriptors: dull, aching, tender, cramping, spasm, hurting, nagging, sickly, sore, twinge, uncomfortable

Neuropathic descriptors: shooting, burning, sharp, smarting, stabbing/dagger-like, tingling, piercing, raw, throbbing, pricking, pins and needles

A wound assessment pain tool has been made available via the internet for clinicians to use during a pain assessment and it includes a body map, pain scales, assessment criteria and suggestions for interventions (Hollinworth, 2005). The author notes that the tool has not been validated, nevertheless, it is a comprehensive instrument for use in clinical practice and, alternatively, it could be used as a reference document for clinicians who wish to update their own tools. It is important to assess wound pain before, during and after the wound care intervention to identify specific pain triggers for the individual.

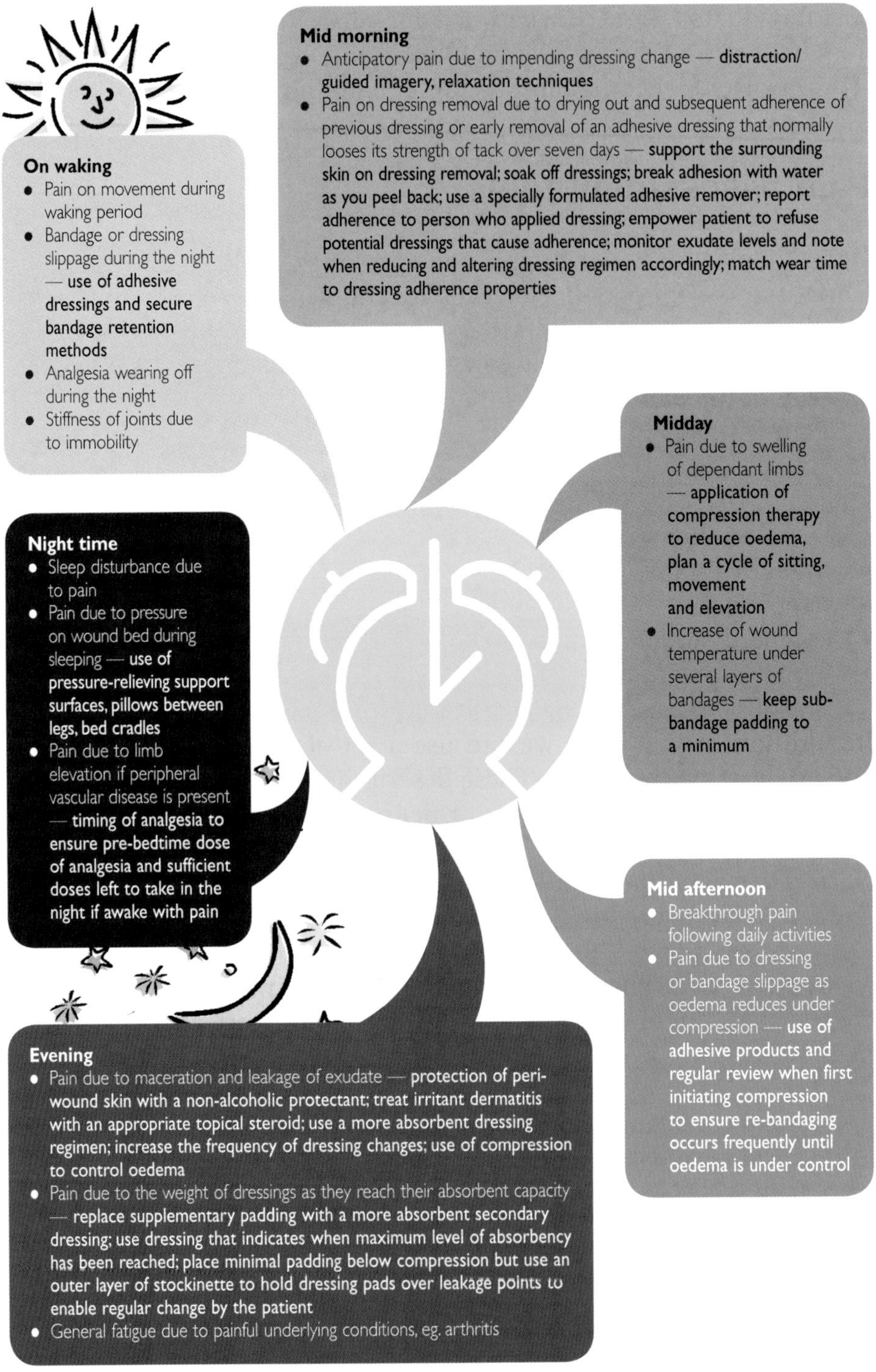

On waking

- Pain on movement during waking period
- Bandage or dressing slippage during the night — **use of adhesive dressings and secure bandage retention methods**
- Analgesia wearing off during the night
- Stiffness of joints due to immobility

Mid morning

- Anticipatory pain due to impending dressing change — **distraction/ guided imagery, relaxation techniques**
- Pain on dressing removal due to drying out and subsequent adherence of previous dressing or early removal of an adhesive dressing that normally looses its strength of tack over seven days — **support the surrounding skin on dressing removal; soak off dressings; break adhesion with water as you peel back; use a specially formulated adhesive remover; report adherence to person who applied dressing; empower patient to refuse potential dressings that cause adherence; monitor exudate levels and note when reducing and altering dressing regimen accordingly; match wear time to dressing adherence properties**

Midday

- Pain due to swelling of dependant limbs — **application of compression therapy to reduce oedema, plan a cycle of sitting, movement and elevation**
- Increase of wound temperature under several layers of bandages — **keep sub-bandage padding to a minimum**

Night time

- Sleep disturbance due to pain
- Pain due to pressure on wound bed during sleeping — **use of pressure-relieving support surfaces, pillows between legs, bed cradles**
- Pain due to limb elevation if peripheral vascular disease is present — **timing of analgesia to ensure pre-bedtime dose of analgesia and sufficient doses left to take in the night if awake with pain**

Mid afternoon

- Breakthrough pain following daily activities
- Pain due to dressing or bandage slippage as oedema reduces under compression — **use of adhesive products and regular review when first initiating compression to ensure re-bandaging occurs frequently until oedema is under control**

Evening

- Pain due to maceration and leakage of exudate — **protection of peri-wound skin with a non-alcoholic protectant; treat irritant dermatitis with an appropriate topical steroid; use a more absorbent dressing regimen; increase the frequency of dressing changes; use of compression to control oedema**
- Pain due to the weight of dressings as they reach their absorbent capacity — **replace supplementary padding with a more absorbent secondary dressing; use dressing that indicates when maximum level of absorbency has been reached; place minimal padding below compression but use an outer layer of stockinette to hold dressing pads over leakage points to enable regular change by the patient**
- General fatigue due to painful underlying conditions, eg. arthritis

Figure 11.4: Pain triggers and reducers

Table 11.3: Pain assessment tools

Type of tool	Advantages	Disadvantages	Client groups
Visual analogue scales	Easy to use	Dependent upon the individual's interpretation of the pain descriptors	Adults and young people

$$0 \qquad\qquad\qquad\qquad 10$$

No pain   Worst pain

Type of tool	Advantages	Disadvantages	Client groups
Numerical rating scale	Easy to use	Person would have to be numerate, sometimes difficult to assign numbers to a dynamic, complex experience	Adults and young people

| 0 | 1 | 2 | 3 | 4 | 5 | 6 | 7 | 8 | 9 | 10 |

No pain   Worst pain

Type of tool	Advantages	Disadvantages	Client groups
Happy faces	Suitable for people that are illiterate or innumerate	May be viewed as childish, the faces may not reflect the individual's cultural ways of expressing pain	Children, people with learning disabilities and those using a different language

Type of tool	Advantages	Disadvantages	Client groups
Coloured ladder	Numeric and literal understanding are not necessary. Helpful when combined with visual analogue and numerical rating scales	Simplistic and thus could cause confusion as a stand-alone ladder	All

Type of tool	Advantages	Disadvantages	Client groups
Verbal rating scale	Uses simple, understandable language	Person would need to be literate	Adults
No pain	Mild pain	Moderate pain	Severe pain

More complex tools, eg. the McGill Pain Questionnaire (Melzack, 1975), allow the individual to scale multiple aspects of the pain experience, whereas the Brief Pain Inventory (Cleeland, 1991) assesses pain and its subjective impact on the individual's activity and functional ability. Nevertheless, both examples are complex and unlikely to be used routinely in clinical practice. It is important that the pain assessment contributes to a pain monitoring system. The following figures and table are examples (*Figures 11.5a, b, 11.6* and *Table 11.4*) of how this can be achieved.

Table 11.4: An example tabular style pain monitoring chart					
Assessment date	Type of pain	Intensity 0–10	Descriptor, eg. stabbing	Reduction goal 0–10	Pain control: analgesia, non-pharmacological methods and dressings
	Background				
	Incident				
	Background				
	Incident				
	Background				
	Incident				

Other pain triggers

There are other pain triggers that may be causing wound pain and we must be alert to these, they may include:

1. The underlying cause of the wound, eg. peripheral vascular disease (*Figure 11.7*).

2. Local factors, for example:
   - wound infection (*Figure 11.8*)
   - irritation caused by varicose eczema
   - dry skin
   - irritant dermatitis
   - desiccation and dryness of the wound bed
   - itching that occurs when a wound is epithelialising

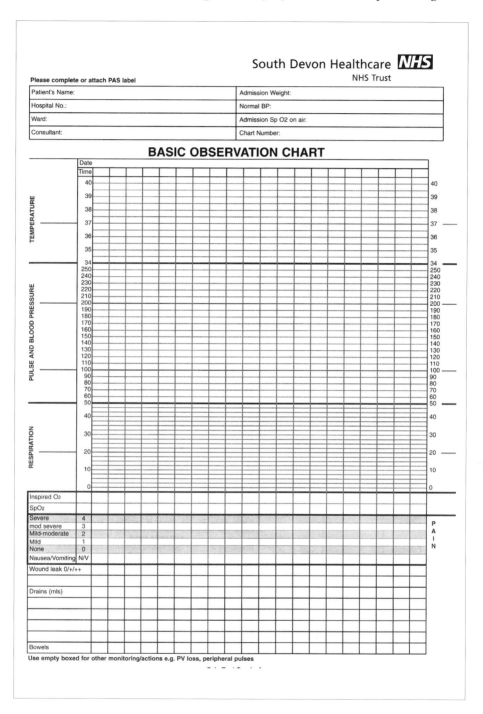

Figure 11.5a: TPR chart with pain monitoring from Torbay Hospital (reproduced with permission). Front side of the chart

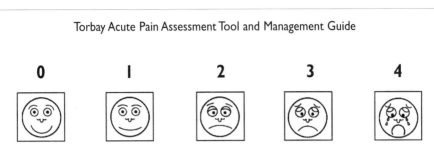

Torbay Acute Pain Assessment Tool and Management Guide

0 1 2 3 4

Pain score all patients at least four hourly
If score ≥ 2 treat as below and recheck every 30 minutes

Pain score	0	1	2	3 and 4
Patients without PCAs or epidurals	Continue regular or PRN analgesia **Paracetamol** 1 g hourly o/PR maximum 4 g/24 hours **Ibuprofen** 400–800 mg orally eight-hourly **Diclofenac** 50 mg O/PR eight-hourly	Continue regular or PRN analgesia	Ensure patient has received paracetamol and NSAID (if not contraindicated). If score remains 2 at 30 minutes consider: **oral morphine** 10 mg or codeine 60 mg or dihydrocodeine 30 mg. If score still 2 at 30 minutes **treat as if 3/4**	Seek help and consider one of the following: 1. **Oral morphine** 10 mg (oromorph or sevredol) 2. **IV morphine** 5–10 mg over 5–10 minutes provided respiration rate > 10 and sedation score ≤ 2 If pain score still 3 or 4 after 30 minutes consider: 3. Repeat dose of O/IV morphine a/a 4. +/- **PCA** 5. Getting an epidural sited Plus ensure patient is receiving regular paracetamol and NSAID (if not contraindicated)
Patients with PCAs	Continue	Continue PCA plus regular oral analgesia	Encourage patient to press PCA button plus regular oral analgesia If score still 2 at 30 minutes treat as if 3/4	Seek help and provided respiration rate > 10 and sedation score ≤ 2 1. Give IV morphine 5–10 mg over 5–10 minutes 2. Encourage patient to press PCA button 3. Ensure patient receives regular oral analgesia If pain score remains 3 or 4 at 30 minutes consider: 4. Repeat IV morphine 5–10 mg over 5–10 minutes 5. Increased bolus doses +/- continuous infusion and **seek help**
Patients with epidurals	Continue	Continue epidural plus regular oral analgesia	Increase rate of epidural infusion plus regular oral analgesia If score still 2 at 30 minutes **treat as if 3/4**	Check epidural site to review catheter position 1. **Seek anaesthetic/APS help for a top up** 2. Increase epidural infusion rate to maximum Plus ensure patient is receiving regular paracetamol and NSAID (if not contraindicated)

Seek help from: your own ward doctors, acute pain service (APS) bleep

Figure 11.5b: Cont. Reverse side of the chart

- swelling due to local inflammation potentially caused by the bacterial load in the wound bed
- pressure or trauma to the wound bed
- uncontrolled oedema.

3. General painful conditions, eg. osteoarthritis (*Figure 11.9*).

4. Anticipatory pain experienced by the individual when they know the dressing change is going to cause them pain. In this situation there is no physical stimulus for the pain, as it is an emotional component of the pain experience (*Figure 11.10*).

Communication

In certain groups of individuals, such as neonates, individuals with confusional states, head injuries, post-cerebral vascular accident or autism, communication may be problematic and we have to rely on non-verbal cues (alteration in posture, facial expressions, bracing, rubbing, guarding, facial contortion, agitation), or changes in the

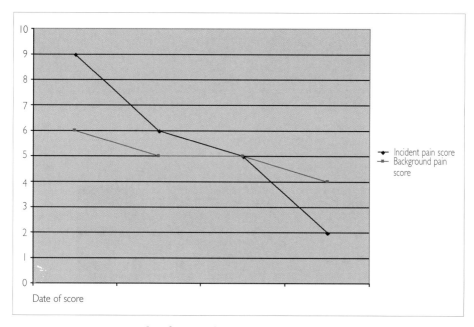

Figure 11.6: An example of a simple pain monitoring line graph using a 0–10 scale (use different colour pens or different connector points, eg. 'x' and 'o')

person's behaviour or alterations in their vital signs. Individuals with learning disabilities may communicate their pain by exhibiting challenging behaviours. A person with dementia may have lost the sense of the geography of their body and consequently cannot indicate the location of their pain (Kerr *et al*, 2006). The disease/condition can affect the motor, cognitive, language and social/emotional capabilities of the individuals to self-report their pain. The traditional pain assessment tools may fail to identify the idiosyncratic pain behaviours that can be characteristic of people with cognitive and neurological impairments. In these situations, the advocate role of the carer is paramount.

In addition, specific patient groups may, as a result of their condition, find themselves experiencing a number of medical and surgical procedures and may be at a higher risk of accidental injury.

We must also remember that pain may be absent in some individuals due to their underlying condition, eg. individuals with spinal injuries or suffering from diabetic neuropathy.

Individuals may harm themselves and produce factitious injuries. It is imperative that we realise that self-injury does not mean a person is insensitive or indifferent to pain.

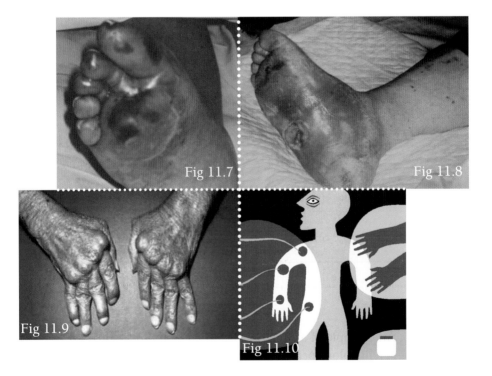

Fig 11.7

Fig 11.8

Fig 11.9

Fig 11.10

Barriers to pain assessment

So far, the assessment of wound pain appears to follow a simple, systematic procedure. However, this is not always the case and there are several factors that hinder or complicate the wound pain assessment process, for example:

- *Age:* this may influence how the person views their pain (cognitive dimension of pain). It may affect the individual's beliefs about their pain and attitudes towards it, eg. displays of stoicism. It can result in mis-attribution of symptoms and the clinician may have to solicit reports of pain. In an elderly population, pain is often attributed to more than one causative factor due to the presence of co-morbidities. The elderly may believe that pain is inevitable and untreatable (Flanagan, 2006).
- *Gender:* this may influence treatment-seeking, delivery of treatment and treatment effectiveness.
- *Culture:* language and ability to express pain may differ between individuals of differing cultures, some being more willing to openly display signs of pain.
- *Being in pain:* this, in itself, can be all-consuming and act as a barrier in the communication process.
- *Nurse/client relationship:* this will be affected by previous experience, trust, acceptance and individual beliefs. A non-judgemental approach is paramount to establishing a therapeutic relationship. Clients will often presume that the clinician is able to take their pain away. The clinician is often the gatekeeper of resources and, therefore, in a very powerful position. Empowerment and shared care can help the client to move along a trajectory towards equality in pain management. Nurses have a professional responsibility to understand, assess and intervene when patients are in pain (Doughty, 2006).
- *Depression:* this may be a predictor of pain severity and induce affective reactions such as feelings of helplessness. This is part of the cognitive dimension of pain which incorporates the emotional impact of the pain on the individual.

Incident pain

Clients with wounds are consistently subjected to dressing changes that may exacerbate the pain generated from their wound. The following quotation should be considered (McQuay *et al*, 1997):

> *Unfortunately, adequate doses are withheld because of traditions, misconceptions, ignorance and fear. Doctors and nurses fear addiction and respiratory depression, but addiction is not a problem with opioid use in acute pain. Opioids given to people who are not in pain or in doses larger than necessary to control the pain can slow or, indeed, stop breathing, irrespective of the route of administration.*

Table 11.5 of pain regimes provides nurses with guidance on how to manage incident pain.

Conclusion

Having considered pain in this chapter we have to acknowledge that its assessment in wounds is multifaceted and consists of verbal reports, non-verbal behaviours and self-reported or observed alterations in daily activities. Individuals rely upon memory for assessment and comparison of pain experiences and this may be absent (in children) or too painful to relive. When assessing wound pain we have to acknowledge the advantages of a rapid, simple assessment using the pain assessment tools, however, these are one-dimensional scales and are unable to assess the complexity of the pain experience. A layered assessment approach that uses variable times and in variable settings will broaden the understanding of the pain experience. It is important to take on guidance from the WUWHS that all wounds are painful and over time they may become more painful, and that, for some clients, even the lightest touch may be excruciatingly painful (WUWHS, 2004). Accepting that their pain is real, even if it appears out of context with the stimulus is vital. It is important to assess wound pain and consequently avoid pain triggers, but rather harness pain reducers into the wound management plan. Nurses need to be professionally competent, knowledgeable and motivated to act in the best interests of their clients, a wealth of knowledge exists that can help to alleviate wound pain for individuals.

This chapter was first published as a Wound Care Society booklet in 2006. It has been modified and is reproduced by kind permission of the Wound Care Society

Table 11.5: Incident pain regimes, pain control regimes 5 and 6

Drug	Dose	Notes
Regime 5. Incident pain (eg. dressing change), based on patient currently taking medication — use all the medications in the regime simultaneously		
Co-codamol 8/500 (8 mg codeine and 500 mg paracetamol, two tables 4–6-hourly	At least 1 hour pre-procedure	Over-the-counter medicine — many trade names, eg. 'Paracodol', 'Solpadeine', 'Panadeine', etc Do not exceed eight tablets in 24 hours Caution when taking other paracetamol containing products Caution in: chronic pancreatitis — see pharmacist or doctor if previously had problems. Liquid or soluble May cause constipation and nausea
Plus		
Ibuprofen 400 mg (one tablet)	At least 1 hour pre-procedure	Many trade names, eg. 'Motrin' 'Nurofen' Caution in: renal disease, GI tract problems, heart failure May cause wheeze and tight chest in asthmatics — seek advice from pharmacist or doctor Take with food. Syrup available
Plus		
Nitrous oxide and oxygen (Entonox)	Inhaled via mouthpiece	Used by patient as required during procedure Good analgesic, it works and wears off quickly Caution in: pneumothorax, intestinal obstruction May be difficult to use in COPD or asthma Some issues regarding transportation and storage in community, so discuss with GP/pharmacist about delivery to the home
Regime 6. Incident pain (eg. dressing change), based on regime 5 being ineffective — use the medications in the regime simultaneously except where it says 'or' then use one of these		
Paracetamol (two tablets)	At least 1 hour pre-procedure	Do not exceed eight tablets in 24 hours Caution if taking other paracetamol containing products Caution in chronic pancreatitis Liquid or soluble available
Plus		
Ibuprofen 400 mg (one tablet)	At least 1 hour pre-procedure	Many trade names, eg. 'Motrin' 'Nurofen' Caution in: Renal disease, GI tract problems, heart failure May cause wheeze and tight chest in asthmatics — seek advice from pharmacist or doctor Take with food. Syrup available
Plus		
Morphine elixir ('Oramorph')	At least 1 hour pre-procedure	Bitter-tasting — it is possible to add blackcurrant cordial to help drinking. May cause nausea and drowsiness

Table 11.5: Cont		
Or Fentanyl lozenge ('Actiq')	As procedure starts	Powerful analgesic, works quickly, lasts for 15 minutes. Initial dose 200 µg — larger doses available Can be used safely in renal impairment
Plus		
Nitrous oxide and oxygen ('Entonox')	Inhaled via mouthpiece	Used by patient as required during procedure Good analgesic as it works and wears off quickly Caution in: pneumothorax, intestinal obstruction
	2 minutes prior to procedure	May be difficult to use in COPD or asthma Some issues regarding transportation and storage in community, so discuss with GP/pharmacist about delivery to the home

Further reading and useful websites

European Wound Management Association (2002) Position Document: *Pain at wound dressing changes*. London: MEP Ltd

Tendra Academy Expert Forum (2006) *Issues in wound care: implementing best practice to minimise trauma and pain*. Tendra Academy, Mölnlycke Health Care, Dunstable

Stevens B, Yamada J, Ohlsson A (2006) *Sucrose for analgesia in newborn infants undergoing painful procedures* (Cochrane review). In: The Cochrane Database of Systematic reviews. Issue 2. Update Software, Oxford

Useful websites:

www.jr2.ox.ac.uk
www.painsociety.org
www.painrelieffoundation.org.uk
www.thepainweb.com
www.pain-talk.co.uk
www.cochrane.org
www.ewma.org
www.tendra.com
www.wuwhs.org
www.worldwidewounds.com
www.nursingceu.com/courses/91/index_nceu.html
www.anaesthesiauk.com

References

Anaesthesia UK (2006) Available online at: www.anaesthesiauk.com/article. aspx?articleid=100118 (last accessed 24 September 2006)

Briggs M, Nelson EA (2004) *Topical agents or dressings for pain in venous leg ulcers* (Cochrane review). In: The Cochrane Library, issue 4. John Wiley & Sons Ltd, Chichester

Cleeland C (1991) Pain Research Group — Used by permission. Available online at: www.caringtotheend.ca/documents/brief_pain_inventory_short.pdf

Doughty D (2006) Strategies for minimizing chronic wound pain. *Adv Skin Wound Care* **19**(2): 82–5

European Wound Management Association (2002) Position Document: *Pain at wound dressing changes*. London: MEP Ltd

Flanagan M (2006) Managing chronic wound pain in primary care. *Practice Nurse* **31**(12): 34–8

Fulgosi D (2006) Available online at: www.medicalmasterclass.com/ pain.%20Fulgosi.htm Concilience Health Resources (last accessed 24 September 2006)

Franks PJ, Moffatt CJ (1998) Who suffers most from leg ulceration? *J Wound Care* **76**(8): 383–5

Hamilton P (2006) Oregon: Pain and pain management. Nursing CEU.com Wild Iris Medical Education. Available online at: www.nursingceu.com/ courses/91/index_nceu.html (last accessed 18 September 2006)

Hollinworth H (2005) *Pain at wound dressing-related procedures: a template for assessment*. Available online at: www.worldwidewounds.com/2005/august/ Hollinworth/Framework-Assessing-Pain-Wound-Dressing-Related.html

IASP Task Force on Taxonomy (2006) Available online at: www.iasp-pain.org/ terms-p.html

Kerr D, Cunningham C, Wilkinson H (2006) *Responding to the pain experiences of older people with a learning difficulty and dementia.* Joseph Rowntree Foundation Communications Department, The Homestead, 40 Water End, York YO30 6WP

Lindholm C, Bjellerup M, Christensen OB, Zederfeldt V (1993) Quality of life in chronic leg ulcer patients: an assessment according to the Nottingham health profile. *Acta Derm Venerol* **73**(6): 440–3

Merskey H, Bogduk (eds) (1994) *Classification of Chronic Pain.* 2nd edn. IASP Press, Seattle. Available online at: www.iasp-pain.org/AM/Template.cfm? Section=Home&template=/CM/HTMLDisplay.cfm&ContentID=4697

McQuay H, Moore A, Justins D (1997) Treating acute pain in hospital. *Br Med J* **314**: 1531–32

McQuay HJ, Dickenson AH (1990) Implications of nervous system plasticity for pain management. *Anaesthesia* **45**: 101–2

Melzack R (1975) The McGill Pain Questionnaire: major properties and scoring methods. *Pain* **1**: 277–99

World Union of Wound Healing Societies (2004) *Principles of best practice: Minimising pain at wound dressing-related procedures*. A consensus document. London: MEP Ltd

Glossary

Allodynia:	Pain due to a stimulus which does not normally provoke pain.
Analgesia:	Absence of pain in response to stimulation which would normally be painful.
Hyperalgesia:	An increased response to a stimulus which is normally painful.
Hypoalgesia:	Diminished pain in response to a normally painful stimulus.
Neuropathic pain:	Pain initiated or caused by a primary lesion, dysfunction, or transitory perturbation in the peripheral or central nervous system.
Nociceptive pain:	Nociceptive pain is mediated by receptors on A-delta and C-fibres. These receptors serve a biologically useful role in localising noxious chemical, thermal and mechanical stimuli. Nociceptive pain can be somatic or visceral in nature. Somatic pain tends to be well localised, constant pain that is described as sharp, aching, throbbing or gnawing. Visceral pain tends to be vague in distribution, paroxysmal in nature and is usually described as deep, aching, squeezing and colicky in nature. Nociceptive pain usually responds to opioids and non-steroidal anti-inflammatory agents.
Nociceptor:	A receptor preferentially sensitive to a noxious stimulus, or to a stimulus which would become noxious if prolonged.
Paresthesia:	An abnormal sensation, whether spontaneous or evoked.

Section III: Scientific developments

CHAPTER 12

THE ISSUE OF BIOFILMS IN WOUNDS

Rose Cooper and Olusola Okhiria

Biofilms are surface-attached microbial communities with characteristic architecture, phenotypic and biochemical properties distinct from their planktonic counterparts. One of the best-known of these biofilm specific properties is the development of antibiotic resistance that can be up to 500-fold greater than that of planktonic cells. Biofilms are not simply a diffusion barrier to resist the action of antimicrobial agents. The greater our understanding of the processes involved in biofilm formation, the greater the chance of developing effective treatment strategies.

There seems to be little doubt that biofilms have the potential to contribute to infection in wounds. To develop strategies to combat wound infections involving biofilms, a greater understanding of the mechanisms of formation and persistence is needed. This chapter will describe biofilm formation and assess its role in human disease and infections. It will also discuss ways biofilms — which are highly resistant to antibiotics — can be targeted.

What is a biofilm?

Complex communities of micro-organisms encased in slime and attached to surfaces are known as biofilms (Costerton *et al*, 1995). They are usually comprised of several different microbial species embedded in sticky extracellular polymers that have been collectively secreted by constituent members. Single species biofilms can be cultivated in the laboratory, but are rare in nature. These structured, functionally co-ordinated communities form on a vast array of living and non-living surfaces and probably represent the commonest form of existence for microbes in natural environments. Conditions that are routinely used in the microbiology laboratory to isolate bacteria from clinical specimens do not, however, generally favour the production of extracellular slimes (known as glycocalyx) (Costerton *et al*, 1978). Therefore, because some biofilm species will not readily grow in cultures and those that do usually fail to produce slime, the presence of biofilms in wounds was not considered until recently. It is likely that the extent of biofilms has been grossly underestimated. The use of poloxamer hydrogels provides an innovative means of encouraging bacteria to exhibit biofilm phenotype in the laboratory and promises to be a valuable laboratory tool to study their behaviour (Percival *et al*, 2007). Another advance is the 'Biofilm Ring Test' for evaluating the ability of bacteria to form biofilms (Chavant *et al*, 2007).

Biofilm formation

Within the past 30 years the development of techniques that provide a means to visualise biofilms in their respective habitats, plus the development of conditions that support the formation and investigation of biofilms in the laboratory, have resulted in a greater understanding of biofilms. Surfaces and interfaces are important in biofilm formation because they facilitate nutrient acquisition. In aquatic environments, nutrients adsorb to surfaces to form a conditioning film with higher concentrations than in bulk solution. Some surfaces (such as dead plants or animals) are themselves a source of nutrients.

Mature biofilms are differentiated, structured communities that reflect complex interactions between microbial cells (Stoodley *et al*, 2002). Some of the species (like *Pseudomonas*) that contribute to biofilms exist in two forms, planktonic (motile) and sessile (non-motile), others (like staphylococci, streptococci and enterococci) are non-motile. Planktonic cells swim and grow as single cells in suspension, whereas cells attracted to a surface can attach and become sessile. Adherence is always the first step towards biofilm development. Attachment (or coaggregation) between different species also leads to the formation of dense microbial aggregates in the early biofilm stages. Attachment is important because it generates intracellular signals that trigger the expression of specific genes essential for biofilm formation and leads to changed phenotypic characteristics (Fegan *et al*, 1990; Li *et al*, 2002).

The synthesis and detection of chemical signals (auto-inducers) facilitates intra-species and inter-species communication, so that relative numbers can be evaluated and the expression of pertinent genes regulated. Cell-to-cell communication via auto-inducers is known as quorum sensing. Many auto-inducers have been discovered, with both discrete and similar molecules in Gram-positive and Gram-negative bacteria; it is probable that many more auto-inducers have yet to be discovered.

Biofilms are diverse and dynamic hydrated structures, constantly changing and adapting to their environment. The developmental stages include reversible and irreversible attachments, followed by phases of maturation and dispersion. Following attachment, microbial cells begin to proliferate into small clusters. When a crucial number is exceeded (sensed by quorum sensing), members excrete extracellular polymeric substances (EPS or matrix) and gradually develop into a biofilm (_Figure 12.1_) (Costerton _et al_, 1999; Sutherland, 2001), while continuing to attract other members — possibly different species of bacteria, fungi, or protozoa (O'Toole _et al_, 2000; Davey and O'Toole, 2000). Extracellular DNA also functions as a glue within a biofilm matrix that helps to stick community members together (Whitechurch _et al_, 2002).

In a mature biofilm, cells embedded in EPS form three-dimensional bulbous, stalked structures that are interspersed with water channels. The water channels act as a crude circulatory or transport system for the movement of nutrients and waste products (Stoodley _et al_, 1994), thereby protecting against starvation by nutrient depletion or inhibition due to the accumulation of toxic metabolites (Davies _et al_, 1998; Sutherland, 2001). Although cells within a biofilm can readily access nutrients and dispose of metabolites, growth rates are always diminished. This confers reduced susceptibility to antimicrobial agents. Cells also exhibit decreased susceptibility to immunological defence mechanisms, particularly phagocytosis, and increased virulence. The close proximity

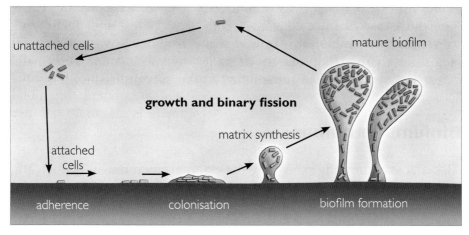

Figure 12.1: Biofilm formation

of organisms within biofilms fosters exchange of genetic material via conjugation and transformation (Hausner and Wuertz, 1999; Wuertz *et al*, 2001), giving the opportunity for organisms with novel combinations of antibiotic resistance and virulence genes to evolve.

Occurrence of biofilms

Biofilms are extensively distributed throughout the natural and industrial world, and their presence may lead to disastrous consequences. About a century ago the discovery of slimes attached to the hulls of ships and boats (now recognised as biofilms), was linked to corrosion. More recently, biofilms have been implicated in the destruction of submerged structures such as oil rigs and piers. Degradation of oil and contamination in wood pulp and paper plants is attributed to biofilms of sulphur bacteria. Biofilms within the lumens of pipelines slow the movement of fluids, cause structural damage by corrosion and present an increased risk of infection. Intermittent release of pathogens such as *Vibrio cholerae* or *Legionella pneumophila* from such pipes in a water distribution system can result in human infection, yet the detection and treatment of such biofilms is problematic because adherent bacteria escape sample collection. Cooling systems associated with ventilated and conditioned air supplies in aeroplanes, hotels and offices similarly can support biofilms, and may be implicated in human infection if not properly maintained. In the home, biofilms occur on the inner surfaces of waste pipes and the wet under-surface of plugs in sinks.

In farming, biofilms have been implicated in animal diseases, such as chronic pneumonia in pigs and mastitis in cows; in plants they cause Pierce's disease of infected grapes and citrus crops, and potato ring rot disease. Some biofilms, however, are beneficial: waste treatment facilities rely on biofilms to degrade organic matter, and metal extraction by leaching in some mining processes utilise biofilms.

Biofilms in humans

All surfaces of the body exposed to the external environment (skin, teeth, oral, respiratory and gastro intestinal epithelia) support a population of sessile, commensal bacteria that possess the ability to form biofilms and yet infection rarely ensues. The majority of such surfaces are constantly being shed, thereby minimising the opportunity of normal species to form biofilms, but slow shedding areas like buccal cavity and the vagina normally sustain biofilm without adverse effects.

Dental plaque is the biofilm that has received the most scientific attention. It was first observed by simple light microscopy during the seventeenth century and is recognised to comprise more than 350 species of bacteria (Moore and Moore, 1994). Biofilms in the mouth, gut, vagina and wounds are not necessarily detrimental and may provide protection against infection (Reid _et al_, 2001).

Biofilms implicated in human disease

It has been estimated that 65% of human infections involve biofilms (Potera, 1999) and this figure may well be too low (Saye, 2007). However, acute infections that are readily treated with antibiotics are not considered to involve biofilms, unlike the majority of chronic infections in mildly compromised individuals that involve commensal or common environmental organisms (Costerton _et al_, 1999). The biofilms most frequently linked to human infection are associated with indwelling medical devices, particularly central venous catheters and protheses. Ingress of micro-organisms on either the exterior or interior surface is possible and infections can be localised to the insertion site, or disseminated to cause bacteraemia, endocarditis or septic shock.

Staphylococcus epidermidis is the most common causative agent associated with implant infections (Rupp and Archer, 1994), but other staphylococcal species, enteric bacteria and _Candida albicans_ have also been implicated. Other devices that have been implicated in biofilm infections include prosthetic heart valves, prosthetic orthopaedic implants, intra-uterine devices, contact lenses, and urinary catheters.

Biofilms associated with implants are a major cause of nosocomial infection. Despite the initially sterile nature of implantable medical devices, inadvertent contamination during insertion, followed by microbial adherence to biomaterials and biofilm initiation can result in unexpected post-operative infection weeks or months after surgery. Dehiscence at the incision site may be the first indication of the problem.

Infections in humans that are linked to biofilms but are not related to devices are typically chronic and difficult to resolve (Costerton _et al_, 1999). They include cystic fibrosis, infectious kidney stones, dental caries, periodontal disease, gingivitis, necrotising fasciitis, chronic prostatitis, osteomyelitis and otitis media (Costerton _et al_, 1999; Parek and Singh, 1999).

Biofilms in wounds

The earliest indication that biofilms may be associated with wounds came from the electron microscopic examination of 15 sutures and 15 staples removed from healed surgical wounds (Gristina et al, 1985). Bacterial cells encased within extracellular material and adherent to the intradermal site of the closures were observed and S. epidermidis was isolated from all of the specimens. These colonised bacteria had caused neither infection nor inflammation, demonstrating that biofilms in humans are not necessarily detrimental. The extracellular material surrounding the bacteria was assumed to have assisted persistence by protecting against host defence mechanisms (Gristina et al, 1985).

The prevalence of biofilms in human cutaneous wounds is not yet established. In one case report, the presence of a biofilm in a chronic leg ulcer of an elderly patient with classic Kaposi sarcoma was suggested. The wound responded only to combined systemic and topical treatment (Boutli-Kasapidou et al, 2006), but the presence of bioflm structures was not confirmed by objective tests such as confocal microscopy.

An Australian research group used light microscopy, confocal laser scanning, electron microscopy and a sophisticated staining technique to confirm that seven out of 12 chronic wounds possessed biofilm (Ngo et al, 2007). They concluded that the necrotic layer on the wound surface appeared to be more conducive to biofilm formation than deeper tissue.

A parallel between biofilms in chronic wounds and cystic fibrosis has been suggested (Bjarnsholt et al, 2007). The presence of large microcolonies of Pseudomonas aeruginosa in chronic wounds was linked to their ability to produce a rhamnolipid that efficiently eliminates polymorphonuclear neutrophils. It was postulated that the inefficient eradication of these opportunist pathogens allowed their persistence and led to the development of biofilms.

Animal models have provided evidence of biofilm formation in acute wounds. In mice, for example, biofilms of Staphylococcus aureus have been demonstrated on silk stitches inserted into skin (Akiyama et al, 1993), and also in croton oil inflamed skin (Akiyama et al, 1994). Electron microscopy of incisions and damaged skin in neutropenic mice that had been inoculated with S. aureus revealed the presence of glycocalyx (Akiyama et al, 1996). Similarly, examination of damaged skin in neutropenic and normal mice by confocal laser scanning microscopy confirmed that inoculated S. aureus produced micro-colonies of cells embedded in glycocalyx (Akiyama *et al*, 2002). Partial-thickness wounds created in three pigs and challenged with *P. aeruginosa* were demonstrated to contain both adherent (EPS positive, hence biofilm producing) and non-adherent bacteria (Serralta *et al*, 2001).

The ability of a clinical isolate of *P. aeruginosa* derived from a burn to grow a biofilm in the laboratory within 10 hours illustrates the potential of wound inhabitants to form biofilm, although *in vitro* (Harrison-Balestra *et al*, 2003). Similarly, *S. aureus* cultures recovered from patients with impetigo, furuncle and atopic dermatitis produced biofilm on coverslips within 72 hours' incubation at 37°C in the presence of plasma, and were deduced to be an inference of biofilms *in vivo* (Akiyama *et al*, 1997).

A porcine model has been utilised to compare the efficacy of antimicrobial agents on planktonic and biofilm phenotypes (Davis *et al*, 2006). Whereas planktonic forms were shown to be eradicated in a relatively short period, established biofilms proved more persistent. The existence of biofilms in diabetic foot ulcers (DFUs) was considered to act as a barrier to effective treatment, as well as causing wound chronicity (Davis *et al*, 2006).

The importance of biofilms in chronic wounds is not yet fully understood, although it has been proposed and discussed (Mertz, 2003). Images and data have been published on the web-site of Montana State University (2006) that suggest a statistically significant association between chronic wounds and biofilms, but none between biofilms and acute wounds. Using scanning electron microscopy and light microscopy of debrided material, biofilms were detected in 30 of 50 chronic wounds, and in one of 16 acute wounds. Given the persistence of some wounds, and their unresponsiveness to antimicrobial agents, it is plausible to attribute chronicity to the presence of biofilms. However, unequivocal evidence has yet to appear in peer-reviewed scientific journals.

Validated methods to detect biofilms in wounds do not yet exist. As stated above, routine investigation of clinical specimens by cultural methods will not normally support glycocalyx synthesis, but occasionally an isolate will simultaneously present as two distinct phenotypes on primary isolation that hint at diversification within the host. *P. aeruginosa*, for example, demonstrating non-mucoid (normal appearance) and mucoid (producing copious amounts of slimy alginate) colonies have been found in a cystic fibrosis patient, indicating biofilm formation (Lam *et al*, 1980).

The presence of slime in a wound does not conclusively indicate the presence of a biofilm, because fibrin deposition is not exclusively mediated by micro-organisms. One indirect indicator of biofilms that has not been explored is the detection of quorum sensing molecules in clinical specimens. Innovative molecular and imaging techniques are being developed for recognising biofilms in joint implants (Stoodley et al, 2005).

Biofilm control

The reduced growth rates of microbial cells within established biofilms confers reduced susceptibility to antimicrobial agents, which in turn contributes to persistence. Additionally, the existence of protected, inactive cells known as persister cells has been proposed (Spoering and Lewis, 2001) and a model to predict survival kinetics has been formulated (Roberts and Stewart, 2005). Organisms residing in biofilms can be more than 500 times less susceptible to antibiotics than planktonic forms (Costerton et al, 1995). The infections associated with biofilms may appear to respond to systemic antibiotics because planktonic cells succumb and symptoms diminish, but persistence of adherent cells leads to recurrent episodes of infection. Two therapeutic approaches to coping with biofilms are possible: prevention and treatment (Table 12.1).

Biofilm prevention

Preventative strategies include blocking bacterial adhesion and interfering with the early events of biofilm initiation and development. It has been suggested that honey can block the formation of Pseudomonas biofilms because molecules of fructose (the most abundant sugar in honey) prevent the bacterium binding to host cell membrane receptor sites and to other bacterial cells (Lerrer et al, 2007). Without adhesion, neither infection nor biofilms develop.

A different approach to disrupting Pseudomonas biofilms has recently been proposed, which relies on changing phenotype with lactoferrin (Singh et al, 2002). Lactoferrin is a constituent of human secretions that is found in tears, mucus and human milk. It can prevent biofilm formation by sequestering iron and stimulating bacteria to adopt a specialised form of motility, which precludes the formation of cell clusters and biofilms. Lactoferrin has also been investigated as a treatment for established biofilms (Davis *et al*, 2006).

Another option that has been considered is to search for molecules that interfere with cell-to-cell communication. The ability to prevent

Table 12.1: Some possible interventions for the management of biofilms

Approach	Strategy	Agent	Microbe(s)	Evidence	Site
Prevention	Interrupt adhesion	Honey	*P. aeruginosa*	*In vitro*	Not tested in wounds
	Prevent adhesion	Lactoferrin	*P. aeruginosa* *S. aureus* *S. epidermidis*	*In vitro* *In vitro* *In vitro*	Clinical trials in DFU ongoing
	Block quorum sensing	Garlic extract	*P. aeruginosa* *P. aeruginosa*	*In vitro* Mouse model	Not tested in wounds, only in lungs
Treatment	Surgical debridement	Scalpel	All species	Theoretical	Not tested in wounds
	Biological debridement	Maggots	All species	Theoretical	Not tested in wounds
	Enzymatic debridement	Mixed enzyme cocktail	All species	Theoretical	Not tested in wounds
	Topical agents	Cadexomer iodine	*S. aureus*	*In vitro*	Not tested in wounds
		Hydrogen peroxide	*S. epidermidis*	*In vitro*	Not tested in wounds
		Povidone iodine	*P. aeruginosa* *S. aureus* *S. epidermidis*	*In vitro* *In vitro* *In vitro*	Not tested in wounds
		Silver	*Candida albicans* *P. aeruginosa* *S. aureus* *S. epidermidis*	*In vitro* *In vitro* *In vitro* *In vitro*	Not tested in wounds
	Electrical destabilisation	Electric current	*S. epidermidis*	*In vitro*	Not tested in wounds
	Infect bacteria with virus	Phage	*P. aeruginosa*	*In vitro* Guinea pig model Mouse model	Burns Burns

or confuse quorum sensing might stop the expression of biofilm and virulence genes. To date no such techniques are available for clinical use, but an extract of garlic that blocked quorum sensing in *P. aeruginosa* made biofilms more susceptible to tobramycin and polymorphonuclear leukocytes. Rapid clearance of lung infections in a mouse model was induced by garlic extract and its potential for treating lung infections in cystic fibrosis patients has been advocated (Bjarnsholt *et al*, 2005). In principle, garlic may be similarly effective in preventing biofilms in wounds.

Compliance with infection control guidelines always helps to minimise infections. In the surgical arena the introduction of strict use of aseptic protocols and filtered laminar air supply in operating theatres reduced the incidence of infection in prosthetic joint surgery (Lidwell *et al*, 1994). Prophylactic and peri-operative antibiotics and the incorporation of antibiotics into bone cement have proved beneficial (Bayston and Milner, 1982), but an increased risk of selecting antibiotic-resistant organisms is possible. Incorporation of antimicrobial agents into and onto implant materials has met with limited success in preventing biofilms. Catheters have been coated with antimicrobial agents, such as antibiotics, antiseptics and silver; antimicrobial agents have also been impregnated into implant materials.

Biofilm treatment

Many treatment methods have been proposed, but none seem ideal. Surgical debridement is thought to be essential for effective control (Costerton *et al*, 1995), so maggots would seem to offer advantages in removing biofilms from wounds. Enzymes have been used to treat biofilms on soft contact lenses (Johansen *et al*, 1997), and promise to be of value in treating wounds (Mertz, 2003).

Antimicrobial agents have not been found to be able to eliminate biofilms from human wounds and *in vitro* evidence to indicate potential efficacy is limited. Four antiseptics were tested *in vitro* against biofilms of *P. aeruginosa* and *Burkholderia cepacia* on Teflon chips. Results showed that 0.2% povidone-iodine effected a 6 log reduction in 10 minutes, whereas inhibition was not detected after 60 minutes exposure to 0.2% solutions of each of chlorhexidine gluconate, benzalkonium chloride or alkyldiaminoethylglycine hydrochloride (Kunisada *et al* 1997). Sucrose in high concentration has induced adverse effects on immature *S. aureus* biofilms, especially in combination with other agents.

Biofilms cultivated on tissue culture coverslips were inhibited by levofloxacin or 10% povidone-iodine together with 70% sucrose and silver sulfadiazine or silver nitrate (Akiyama *et al*, 1998). In both of the above studies, cell counts were used to monitor biofilm changes; another approach has been to observe changes using microscopy. Confocal laser scanning microscopy was used to determine the effect of cadexomer iodine on *S. aureus* biofilms *in vivo* and *in vitro* (Akiyama *et al*, 2004). Bacterial cells surrounded by glycocalyx were located among cadexomer iodine beads, suggesting that biofilm structures were destroyed, glycocalyx was reduced by dehydration and that bacteria were killed. Inhibition of *S. epidermidis* biofilms by alcohols, povidone-iodine and hydrogen peroxide has also been investigated (Presterl *et al*, 2007).

Atomic force microscopy and scanning electron microscopy were utilised to measure disruption of *S. epidermidis* biofilms by silver ions (Chaw *et al*, 2005). Whereas the viability of sessile cells was not affected by 60 minutes contact with low concentrations of silver ions (50 ppb), biofilm integrity was markedly impaired. Measurements showed that silver ion treatment reduced intermolecular forces in extracellular polymeric substances (EPS). The authors suggested that the binding of highly reactive silver ions to electron donor groups of matrix components prevented them forming electrostatic hydrogen bonds and divalent cation bridges that normally stabilise a biofilm matrix. Biofilm destabilisation resulted (Chaw *et al*, 2005). Although the concentration of silver ions used in this study was not inhibitory, the ability to disrupt biofilms may stimulate the development of novel strategies for clinical situations in the future.

Antimicrobial effects of two silver dressings have been studied using the poloxamer gel model (Percival *et al*, 2007) and different efficacies were reported. The principle of destabilising biofilms with electric current has been suggested for *S. epidermidis* on surgical stainless steel (Van der Borden *et al*, 2004a). Newly-adhered staphylococci were stimulated to detach from surfaces by application of direct or block current > 100 μA, but direct current was more effective than block current in treating a growing *S. epidermidis* biofilm (Van der Borden *et al*, 2004b).

One novel approach to treating bacterial infections that has some potential with biofilms is the use of bacterial viruses (or phages). This therapy has been used successfully in Georgia for many years. It relies on establishing a viral infection in a bacterial pathogen and results in bacterial death and lysis, which eradicates the pathogen from the patient without side-effects. To date, most of the research has been conducted in burns. Using guinea pigs experimentally infected with lethal doses of *P. aeruginosa*, the ability of pseudomonas phage to prevent skin graft rejection in six out of seven cases was observed, whereas all untreated grafts failed (Soothill, 1994). Decreased mortality rates in a mouse burn model using pseudomonas phages have also been reported (McVay *et al*, 2007). The ultimate success of this strategy will depend on employing the specific strain of viruses for each strain of pathogen.

Conclusion

The existence of polymicrobial communities in wounds is not unexpected (Bowler *et al*, 2001). Although biofilms are not yet routinely characterised in human wounds, there seems to be little doubt that they have the potential to contribute to infections and persistence. Effective treatment strategies are essential, and the better that the processes involved in biofilm formation are understood, the greater is the chance of developing appropriate remedies. There have been many developments in the past few years, but there is still some way to go.

References

Akiyama H, Torigoe R, Arata J (1993) Interaction of *Staphylococcus aureus* cells and silk threads *in vitro* and in mouse skin. *J Dermatol Sci* 6: 247–57

Akiyama H, Kanazaki H, Tada J, Arata J (1994) *Staphylococcus aureus* infection on cut wounds in the mouse skin: experimental botryomycosis. *J Dermatol Sci* 8: 1–10

Akiyama H, Kanazaki H, Tada J, Arata J (1996) *Staphylococcus aureus* infection on experimental croton oil-inflamed skin in mice. *J Dermatol Sci* 11: 234–8

Akiyama H, Huh W-K, Yamasaki O, Oono T, Iwatsuki K (2002) Confocal laser scanning microscopic observation of glycoclayx production by *Staphylococcus aureus* in mouse skin: does *S. aureus* generally produce a biofilm on damaged skin? *Br J Dermatol* 147: 879–85

Akiyama H, Oono T, Saito M, Iwatsuki K (2004) Assessment of cadexomer iodine against *Staphylococcus aureus* biofilm *in vivo* and *in vitro* using confocal laser scanning microscopy. *J Dermatol* 31: 529–34

Akiyama H, Torigoe R, Arata J (1993) Interaction of _Staphylococcus aureus_ cells and silk threads _in vitro_ and _in vivo_ and in mouse skin. _J Dermatol Sci_ **6**: 247–57

Akiyama H, Ueda M, Kanazaki H, Tada J, Arata J (1997) Biofilm formation of _Staphylococcus aureus_ strains isolated from impetigo and furuncle: role of fibrinogen and fibrin. _J Dermatol Sci_ **16**: 2–10

Akiyama H, Yamasaki O, Kanzaki H, Tada J, Arata J (1998) Effects of sucrose and silver on _Staphylococcus aureus_ biofilms. _J Antimicrob Chemother_ **42**: 629–34

Bayston R, Milner RDC (1982) The sustained release of antimicrobial drugs from bone cement. _J Bone Joint Surg_ **64B**: 460–4

Bjarsholt T, Jensen PØ, Rasmussen TB, _et al_ (2005) Garlic blocks quorum sensing and promotes rapid clearance of pulmonary _Pseudomonas aeruginosa_ infections. _Microbiology_ **151**: 3873–89

Bjarnsholt T, Kirketerp-Møller K, Østrup Jenson P, _et al_ (2007) Why chronic wounds will not heal: a novel hypothesis. _Wound Rep Regen_ **11**: 1–9

Boutli-Kasapidou B, Delli F, Avgoustinaki N, Lambrou N, Tsatsos M, Karakatsanis G (2006) What are biofilms? Evaluation and management in open skin wounds. _Eur Acad Dermatol Venereol_ **20**(6): 743–5

Bowler PG, Duerden BI, Armstrong DG (2001) Wound microbiology and associated approaches to wound management. _Clin Microbiol Rev_ **14**(2): 244–69

Chaw KC, Manimaran M, Tay FEH (2005) Role of silver ions in destabilization of intermolecular adhesion forces measured by atomic force microscopy in _Staphylococcus epidermidis_ biofilms. _Antimicrob Agents Chemother_ **49**(12): 4853–9

Chavant P, Gaillard-Martinie B, Talon R, _et al_ (2007) A new device for rapid evaluation of biofilm formation potential by bacteria. _J Micro Meth_ **68**: 605–12

Costerton JW, Geesey GG, Cheng KJ (1978) How bacteria stick. _Sci Am_ **238**(1): 86–95

Costerton JW, Lewandowski Z, Caldwell DE, Korber DR, Lappin-Scott HM (1995) Microbial biofilms. _Annu Rev Microbiol_ **49**: 711–45

Costerton JW, Stewart PS, Greenberg EP (1999) Bacterial biofilms: a common cause of persistent infections. _Science_ **284**: 1318–22

Davey ME, O'Toole GA (2000) Microbial biofilms: from ecology to molecular genetics. _Microbiol Mole Biol Rev_ **64**(4): 847–67

Davies DG, Parsek MR, Pearson JP, Iglewski BH, Costerton JW (1998) The involvement of cell-to-cell signals in the development of a bacterial biofilm. _Science_ **280**: 295–8

Davis SC, Martinez L, Kirsner R (2006) The diabetic foot: the importance of biofilms and wound bed preparation. *Curr Diabetes Reports* **6**(6): 439–46

Fegan M, Francis P, Hayward AC, Davis GH, Fuerst JA (1990) Phenotypic conversion of *Pseudomonas aeruginosa* in cystic fibrosis. *J Clin Microbiol* **28**(6): 1143–6

Gristina AG, Price JL, Hobgood CD, Webb LX, Costerton JW (1985) Bacterial colonization of percutaneous sutures. *Surgery* **98**(1): 12–19

Harrison-Balestra C, Cassaniga AL, Davis SC, Mertz PM (2003) A wound-isolated *Pseudomonas aeruginosa* grows a biofilm *in vitro* within 10 hours and is visualized by light microscopy. *Dermatol Surg* **29**(6): 631–5

Hausner M, Wuertz S (1999) High rates of conjugation in bacterial biofilms as determined by quantitative in situ analysis. *Appl Environ Microbiol* **65**(8): 3710–13

Johansen C, Falholt P, Gram (1997) Enzymatic removal and disinfection of bacterial biofilms. *Appl Environ Microbiol* **63**(9): 3724–28

Kunisada T, Yamada K, Oda S, *et al* (1997) Investigation on the efficacy of povidone-iodine against antiseptic-resistant species. *Dermatol* **195**(suppl 2): 14–18

Lam J, Chan R, Lam K, Costerton JW (1980) Production of mucoid microcolonies by *Pseudomonas aeruginosa* within infected lungs in cystic fibrosis patients. *Infect Immun* **28**(2): 546–56

Lerrer Lerrer B, Zinger-Yosovitch KD, Avrahami B, Gilboa-Garber N (2007). Honey and royal jelly, like human milk, abrogate lectin-dependent infection-preceding *Pseudomonas aeruginosa* adhesion. *ISME J* **1**: 149–55

Li YH, Tang N, Aspiras MB, Lau PC, Lee JH, Ellen RP, Cvitkovitch DG (2002) A quorum-sensing signalling system essential for genetic competence in Streptococcus mutans is involved in biofilm formation. *J Bacteriol* **184**(10): 2699–708

Lidwell OM, Lowbury EJL, Whyte W, Blowers R, Stanley SJ, Lowe R (1984) Infection and sepsis after operations for total hip or knee-joint replacement: influence of ultraclean air, prophylactic antibiotics and other factors. *J Hygiene* **93**: 505–29

McVay CS, Velásquez M, Fralick JA (2007) Phage therapy of *Pseudomonas aeruginosa* in a mouse burn wound model. *Antimicrob Agents Chemother* **51**(6): 1934–8

Mertz PM (2003) Cutaneous biofilms: friend or foe? *Wounds* **15**(5): 129–32

Montana State University (2006) Biofilm control collection. Available online at: www.erc.montana.edu/Res-Lib99-SW/Image_Library/Biofilm_Control/default.htm (last accessed 31 May, 2006)

Moore WE, Moore LV (1994) The bacteria of periodontal diseases. *Peridontology* **5**: 66–77

Ngo Q, Vickery K, Deva AK (2007) Role of bacterial biofilms in chronic wounds. *Aust N Z J Surg* 77(suppl 1): A66

O'Toole, G, Kaplan HB, Kolter R (2000) Biofilm formation as microbial development. *Annu Rev Microbiol* 54: 49–79

Percival SL, Bowler PG, Dolman J (2007) Antimicrobial activity of silver-containing dressings on wound micro-organisms using an *in vitro* biofilm model. *Int Wound J* 4(2): 186–191

Potera C (1999) Forging a link between biofilms and disease. *Science* 283: 1837–9

Presterl E, Suchomel M, Eder M, *et al* (2007) Effects of alcohols, povidone-iodine and hydrogen peroxide on biofilms of *Staphylococcus epidermidis*. *J Antimicrob Chemother* 60: 417–20

Reid G, Howard J, Bing SG (2001) Can bacterial interference prevent infection? *Trends Microbiol* 9(9): 424–8

Roberts ME, Stewart PS (2005) Modelling protection from antimicrobial agents in biofilms through the formation of persister cells. *Microbiology* 151: 75–80

Rupp ME, Archer GL (1994) Coagulase-negative staphylococci: pathogens associated with medical progress. *Clin Infect Dis* 19: 231–45

Saye DE (2007) Recurring and anti-microbial-resistant infections: considering the potential role of biofilms in clinical practice. *Ostomy/Wound Management* 53(4): 46–62

Serralta VW, Harrison-Belestra C, Cazzaniga AL, Davis SC, Mertz PM (2001) Lifestyles of bacteria in wounds: presence of biofilms? *Wounds* 13(1): 29–34

Singh PK, Parsek MR, Greenberg EP, Welsh MJ (2002) A component of innate immunity prevents bacterial biofilm development. *Nature* 41 (6888): 552–5

Soothill JS (1994) Bacteriophage prevents destruction of skin grafts by *Pseudomonas aeruginosa*. *Burns* 20: 209–11

Spoering AL, Lewis K (2001) Biofilms and planktonic cells of *Pseudomonas aeruginosa* have similar resistance to killing by antimicrobials. *J Bacteriol* 183: 6746–51

Stoodley P, Debeer D, Lewandowsky Z (1994) Liquid flow in biofilm systems. *Appl Environ Microbiol* 60(8): 2711–6

Stoodley P, Sauer K, Davies DG, Costerton JW (2002) Biofilms as complex differentiated communities. *Annu Rev Microbiol* 56: 187–209

Stoodley P, Kathju S, Hu FZ, *et al* (2005) Molecular and imaging techniques for bacterial biofilms in joint arthroplasty infections. *Clin Orthop Rel Res* 437: 31–40

Sutherland IW (2001) The biofilm matrix – an immobilised but dynamic microbial environment. *Trends Microbiol* 9(5): 222–7

Van der Borden AJ, van der Werf H, van der Mei C, Busscher HJ (2004a) Electric current-induced detachment of *Staphylococcus epidermidis* biofilms from surgical stainless steel. *Appl Environ Microbiol* **70**(11): 6871–4

Van der Borden AJ, van der Werf H, van der Mei C, Busscher HJ (2004b) Electric current-induced detachment of *Staphylococcus epidermidis* biofilms from surgical stainless steel. *J Biomed Materials Res* **68B**: 160–4

Whitechurch CB, Tolker-NielsenT, Ragas PC, Mattick JS (2002) Extracellular DNA required for biofilm formation. *Science* **295**: 1487

Wuertz S, Hendrickx L, Kuehn M, Rodenacker K, Hausner M (2001) In situ quantification of gene transfer in biofilms. *Methods Enzymol* **336**: 129–43

CHAPTER 13

FACTORS INVOLVED IN CRITICAL COLONISATION OF CHRONIC WOUNDS

Richard White and Keith Cutting

Infection in chronic wounds presents a major clinical challenge and is a cause of high morbidity. Much attention has been given to identifying and managing this problem since the publication of the seminal article on chronic wound infection criteria (Cutting and Harding, 1994). Those pathogenic micro-organisms which cause wound infection have first to overcome a wide range of specific and non-specific antimicrobial mechanisms, and, phagocytic cells (polymorphonuclear neutrophils or PMNs) which form a crucial part of the innate host response against bacterial infection (Kobayashi *et al*, 2003). Invading bacteria become opsonised by complement proteins or antibodies and subsequently phagocytosed and killed by PMNs. To illustrate how alteration in wound bioburden impacts pathology, the Wound Infection Continuum (WIC) has been devised and subsequently modified (Gray *et al*, 2005). One stage in this continuum, critical colonisation, is putatively described as a pivotal phase that occurs without inducing an overt host response. Critical colonisation is better explained from a microbiological than from a clinical perspective. The status of critically colonised wounds may change in one of several ways: 1) deteriorate to clinical infection, 2) remain in a critically colonised state, or 3) improve following appropriate intervention. Research to clearly define the term and clarify the role of bioburden in the chronic wound is needed to help clinicians recognise and implement appropriate treatment.

The term critical colonisation has attracted increasing attention over the past five years. It has been regarded by a number of authors as synonymous with local infection (Schultz *et al*, 2003; Edwards and Harding, 2004; Jorgenson *et al*, 2004; Sibbald *et al*, 2004) through its association with the criteria for wound infection developed by Cutting and Harding (1994), a benchmark for diagnosis that appears to have gained relatively broad acceptance. Some have dismissed the concept of critical colonisation as a myth, expressing the view that a wound is either infected or not, with no prodromal phase of infection (Gilchrist, 2003). In order to advance understanding of delayed healing in the absence of an obvious clinical cause, the basic concept of critical colonisation deserves consideration.

If alternative explanations for delayed healing can be identified, patient morbidity potential can be reduced. Delayed healing must be placed accurately into context to help avoid making or perpetuating inappropriate assumptions. This chapter reviews the emergence of the concept of critical colonisation from an historical perspective, discusses assumptions that have been made, and presents scientific evidence collated from the literature. This approach draws some parallels with the criteria for wound infection developed by Cutting and Harding (1994), where a review of the literature led to the collation of traditional and additional diagnostic features of wound infection and the development of an entirely new approach to identifying clinical wound infection. These criteria, later validated by Cutting (1998), have been refined by Cutting and White, 2005.

Development of the concept

The term critical colonisation was first coined in 1996 by Davis in a poster presented to a joint meeting of the Wound Healing Society (WHS) and the European Tissue Repair Society (ETRS). Using case studies, Davis demonstrated how delayed healing in wounds could be reversed through appropriate use of topical antiseptics. She also defined the condition of the wound in relation to bacterial presence. Using a modified model for infection first published by Ayton (1985), Davis introduced the notion of critical colonisation within the infection spectrum (from sterile to contaminated to colonised to critically colonised to infection) and defined it as 'multiplication of organisms without invasion but interfering with wound healing.' Davis also stated that 'the classic signs of infection must be reassessed to include the "critically colonised" wound,' (1996) offering the first association with local infection. In support of her treatise, Davis cited Danielson (1994) and a clinical study with microbiological screening by Trengove et al (1996), espousing the notion that the presence of pathogens, with or without host reaction, could interfere with healing. Currently, the absence of a host response is viewed as a fundamental link to understanding the concept of critical colonisation. Davis continued to champion the term critical colonisation, but little, if any notice was taken until Kingsley (2001) renamed her model of wound infection 'the Wound Infection Continuum'. This model is most closely associated with chronic wounds, where sterility and contamination are not clinically relevant and colonisation may be regarded as the 'normal' state.

While the term critical colonisation may sound novel, the underpinning concept has been part of the wound healing

Table 13.1: Critical colonisation: factors involved in delayed healing

- Immuno-invasion
- Apoptosis
- Anti-inflammatory and anti-angiogenic
- Biofilm formation
- Cytotoxicity
- Chronic inflammation (*Figure 13.1*)
- Trojan horse

lexicon under various guises. A review of the literature in relation to delayed healing reveals the use of a number of synonymous phrases, including silent infection, covert infection (Dow, 2003), occult infection (Sibbald *et al*, 2003), refractory wound (Markus *et al*, 2006), subclinical infection (Hermanns *et al*, 1999), indolent wound (Kingsley, 2003), stunned wound (Ennis and Menenses, 2000), sub-acute infection, and recalcitrant wound (Selkon *et al*, 2006).

Critical colonisation in clinical context

Role in the Wound Infection Continuum

With heightened focus on wound microbiology and infection in recent years, the Wound Infection Continuum has been proposed as a model to account for an increasing microbial load (bioburden) and related pathology (Kingsley, 2001; 2003). Although the concept of critical colonisation is not universally accepted, clinicians and researchers generally agree that the term needs definitive characterisation in order to validate its consideration in infection management (Ovington, 2003; Cutting and White, 2005).

Wound infection development depends on complex microbial and host factors with the latter being the governing factor. While many will claim quantitative bacterial values as a criterion for infection, the reliance on numbers is unjustified in chronic wounds (Bowler, 2003).

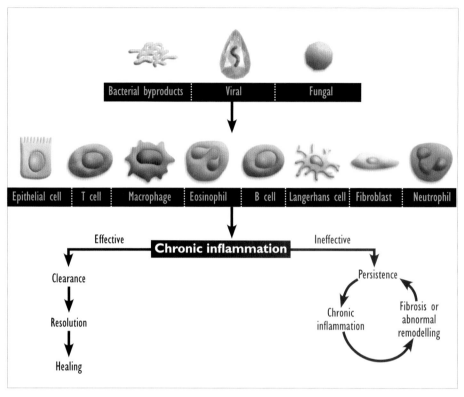

Figure 13.1: The influence of infectious agents on chronic wound inflammation and delayed healing

An *in vivo* study (Trengove *et al*, 1994) has shown that the number of bacterial species and the number of organisms are important factors in the development of infection. However, these findings have yet to be clinically validated. In a theoretical hypothesis, Heinzelmann *et al* (2002) submit that the host response, or immune status of the individual, is a key factor in the development of infection; the triggering of a host response has been used as a diagnosis of infection for 2000 years.

For those who accept it as a distinct entity, critical colonisation is a stage where wound healing is delayed by microbial factors without the overt signs and symptoms of infection (Cutting, 2003); it occurs despite optimum treatment (Kingsley, 2003). It would appear to be a contradiction that a microbially induced delay in healing could occur without eliciting a host response. How could such a situation arise without the host response playing a part? A number of authors have reported delayed ulcer healing influenced by micro-organisms: Lookingbill *et al* (1978) in a quantitative bacteriology study on 13 leg ulcers; Daltrey *et al* (1981) in a bacteriological study of 74 pressure ulcers in 53 patients; Halbert *et al* (1992) in a bacteriological study of 82 patients with 100 ulcerated limbs; and Hansson *et al* (1995) in a study of the qualitative and quantitative bacteriology of 58 patients with leg ulcers. In a retrospective review of patients with various inflammatory wounds such as *necrobiosis lipoidica*, Drosou *et al* (2003) provide an additional perspective, stating it is likely that subclinical damage to tissue as a result of bacterial contamination exists and cites Hermanns *et al* (1999) in support of this premise.

Clinically, host response to wound infection is recognised by the classic signs and symptoms of inflammation, ie. redness, swelling, warmth, and pain. Spreading erythema around the wound is usually indicative of infection such as erysipelas or cellulitis (Hansson *et al*, 1995). However, not all erythematous reactions are immunologically generated. Recent findings from a series of clinical cases have shown that Morganella species (notably *M. morganii*) commonly found in wounds express histamine in physiologically significant amounts (Cooper *et al*, 2004); therefore, in some wounds periwound erythema could be attributable to *M. morganii* colonisation. This Gram-negative bacillus inhabits the gastro-intestinal tract and is a part of the normal faecal flora. It has been reported in chronic leg ulceration (Aspiroz *et al*, 2004) and in Chiclero's ulcer in a microbiological study involving 26 patients (Aspiroz *et al*, 2004), but is not routinely considered in bacterial samples acquired from wounds. Hansson *et al* (1995) found *M. morganii* (identified as *Proteus morganii*) in 23% of venous leg ulcers (n = 58) studied. Conversely, Bowler and Davies (1999), in a review of data from a prospective clinical study where swabs from 44 infected leg ulcers were compared with 30 from non-infected ulcers, found this bacterium in 'infected' but not 'non-infected' leg ulcers. In this study, the diagnosis of ulcer infection was determined on the basis of clinical signs including erythema, cellulitis, oedema, increased pain, increased exudate, and warmth.

Microbial factors

In literature reviews of the cell biology of chronic wounds, delayed healing has been intimately linked with uncontrolled inflammation (Meneghin and Hogaboam, 2007; Eming *et al*, 2007; Menke *et al*, 2007) or immunopathology (Page *et al*, 2006). This is not visually evident in many chronic wounds because it is not always accompanied by the classical signs of inflammation. However, delayed healing is histologically evident (Abd-El-Aleem *et al*, 2005). The acolytes of critical colonisation believe delayed healing often can be attributed to microbial factors (Gray *et al*, 2005), and that frequently diagnosis is confirmed only retrospectively once antimicrobial measures have been taken and found to be effective.

How, then, can delayed healing be associated with microbial factors and not elicit an obvious host response? Three or more potential bacterial modes of action, described in the literature, can delay wound healing without any apparent inflammatory or immunological response: the expression of immuno-evasion (Allen *et al*, 2005), biofilm formation (Serralta *et al*, 2001; *Chapter 12*), and suppression of cellular wound healing responses (Stephens *et al*, 2003). These modes have been identified following *in vitro* work and can occur when the wound is colonised by certain specific bacteria.

Pseudomonas aeruginosa

An organism commonly found in chronic wounds (Bowler and Davies, 1999) and associated with chronic infection (Lau *et al*, 2004), *Pseudomonas aeruginosa* is known to form biofilms (Costerton, 2001) and secrete immuno-evasive factors (Usher *et al*, 2002) active against polymorphonucleocytes (PMNs). To this effect, activation of the type III secretion system, a recently identified virulence determinant of *P. aeruginosa*, has been reported from *in vitro* studies using clinical isolates (Dacheux *et al*, 2002). It has been postulated from *in vitro* studies that *P. aeruginosa* is likely to be of far greater significance to wound chronicity, tissue invasion, and infection than previously recognised (Serralta *et al*, 2001; King *et al*, 2003; Stephens *et al*, 2003; Allen *et al*, 2005; White, 2006).

As indicated in a summary of clinical and microbiology findings by Hamilton and Danielsen (1997), experienced wound clinicians have long noticed occasional green colouration in chronic wounds and have associated it with the presence of *P. aeruginosa* and delayed healing. Green wounds have been diagnosed as infected on the basis of colour alone (Benbow, 2007). This we now know to be inaccurate. The green pigment, pyocyanin, is a phenazine, a highly diffusible exotoxic metabolite described in an *in vitro* study by Denning *et al* (2003). In a review of published clinical and *in vitro* data by Lau *et al* (2004), pyocyanin has been shown to inhibit many cell functions and impair host defences through apoptosis. *In vitro* laboratory research on clinical samples (Zychlinsky and Sansonetti, 1997a) has shown that many pathogens, including *P. aeruginosa*, induce inappropriate or premature apoptosis (programmed cell death) of immune cells such as macrophages and neutrophils and that this can be pro-inflammatory (Zychlinsky and Sonsonetti, 1997b).

P. aeruginosa has evolved immuno-evasive strategies by which it affects host immunity (Buret and Cripps, 1993). *In vitro* studies have shown pyocyanin and other similar phenazines to have pro-apoptotic action on human neutrophils (Usher *et al*, 2002). This is postulated to be a clinically important mechanism of persistence of *P. aeruginosa* in human tissue (Usher *et al*, 2002). What mediates the change in the infective potential of this organism? *P. aeruginosa* has been shown in a literature review to be a phenotypically unstable pathogen, particularly in chronic infection (Speert, 2002). The virulence of *P. aeruginosa* is controlled by an N-acyl homoserine lactone (AHL)-dependent quorum sensing system. The organism has been shown *in vitro* to have the capability to modulate its own quorum-sensing dependent pathogenic potential through an AHL-acylase enzyme (Sio *et al*, 2006). This may in part explain how under certain circumstances *P. aeruginosa* may be a delayer of wound healing and under other circumstances an infecting organism.

A parallel has been drawn between the chronicity of some wounds (venous leg ulcers, pressure ulcers, and diabetic foot ulcers) and cystic fibrosis (Bjarnsholt *et al*, 2007) insofar as *P. aeruginosa* is implicated in biofilm formation, polymorphonuclear neutrophil function, and a possible 'shielding' mechanism which protects the bacterium from phagocytosis (Jensen *et al*, 2006; Bjarnsholt *et al*, 2005). The authors postulate that 'the presence of *P. aeruginosa* in biofilms, and the lack of concomitant elimination by attended PMNs, are the main causes of inefficient eradication by antibiotic treatment and antimicrobial activity of the innate immune system, respectively' (Bjarnsholt *et al*, 2007). While this article relates to what the authors describe as 'infection in chronic wounds', it will apply equally to what has been described as 'critical colonisation'. Furthermore, in cystic fibrosis, *P. aeruginosa* is found with *Burkholderia cepacia*, possibly in symbiosis or synergy. This situation could be the case in chronic wounds where the synergy becomes one virulence determinant of many.

Other aerobes and anaerobes also have been recognised for down-regulating the immune response. In an *in vitro* microbiology study, Bowler *et al* (1999) summarised the role of succinate (a dicarboxylic acid) produced by aerobes and anaerobes; *in vitro* studies by Rotstein *et al* (1987; 1989) demonstrate how succinate may increase the risk of infection by impairing host cell function.

Escherichia coli is both a normal member of the intestinal flora, and, a prominent human pathogen causing a broad spectrum of diseases. It is routinely found in chronic wounds such as sacral pressure ulcers and venous leg ulcers (Bowler and Davies, 1999; Brook and Frazier, 1998). A mechanism whereby *E.coli* subverts the innate immune system has recently been described (Fexby *et al*, 2007). A surface protein on *E.coli* — antigen 43 (Ag43) — has been shown to promote bacterial binding to some human cells, biofilm formation, enhanced resistance towards antibacterial agents, and, the capacity to survive phagocytosis by PMNs in an opsonin-independent manner, in effect a 'Trojan horse' (Fexby *et al*, 2007). While this has yet to be demonstrated in wounds, it may provide part of the rationale for 'chronic' inflammation and for critical colonisation.

Staphylococcus aureus

Staphylococcus aureus is also an important human wound pathogen that interferes with host-cell functions. According to *in vitro* studies, impaired healing often is observed in *S. aureus*-infected wounds where the extracellular adherence protein (EAP) has been implicated (Athanasopoulos *et al*, 2006). Extracellular adherence protein has been shown in *in vitro* studies to be a potent anti-inflammatory (Chavakis *et al*, 2002) and anti-angiogenic agent, preventing recruitment of inflammatory cells to the wound site as well as inhibiting neovascularisation (Haggar *et al*, 2004).

Odour-producing micro-organisms

Wound malodour, a common characteristic of chronic wounds, has been linked to short-chain fatty acids (SCFAs) in *in vitro* studies (Bowler *et al*, 1999). These volatile compounds are the metabolic by-products of anaerobic bacterial metabolism. Malodour is associated with organisms known to generate SCFAs such as *Bacteroides spp* and anaerobic cocci (Haggar *et al*, 2004). In an *in vitro* study, Stephens *et al* (2003) demonstrated that Peptostreptococci-generated SCFA inhibited the growth of key cells responsible for wound healing, eg. keratinocytes, fibroblasts, and endothelial cells. If translated to the *in vivo* situation, this could result in delayed healing from uncomplicated colonisation (ie. no perceived clinical or cellular effects) without the bioburden necessarily reaching a theoretical infection threshold. Hansson *et al*'s *in vivo* study (1995) found Peptostreptococcus species (identified as *P. magnus*, *P. asaccharolyticus* and *P. prevotii*) in 30% of venous leg ulcers. This is a clinically significant level of species-specific colonisation and indicates the importance of anaerobic involvement in chronic wound bacteriology.

Short-chain fatty acids studies *in vitro* have been shown to play a part in impairing neutrophil chemotaxis and phagocytosis (Stephens *et al*, 2003). The low pH of all chronic wounds facilitates succinate activity and provides a milieu that down-regulates neutrophil function (Rotstein *et al*, 1987; 1989).

Differentiating critical colonisation as a distinct stage of infection

From the theses presented, it can be observed that a chronic wound colonised but not infected with one or more of certain bacteria (among them *Morganella spp*, *P. aeruginosa* and *Peptostreptococcus spp*) may exhibit erythema and delayed healing without a traditional or otherwise evident host response. Scenarios involving these organisms and possibly others yet to be identified have been used to postulate the concept of critical colonisation.

The critical nature of colonisation takes on a far greater significance when viewed in this light. A low level of colonisation may be all that is required to delay healing and is far removed from that required for local infection to be diagnosed in terms of the level of bioburden and the demonstration of signs of infection (host response). The clinical indicators of infection developed by Cutting and Harding (1994) (and validated by Cutting [1998] a few years later regarding the decisions made by nurses on the infection state of a variety of wounds) should remain firmly aligned within the domain of local infection. Simply renaming local infection as critical colonisation has no value (Bowler, 1998).

The fundamental message is that a number of possible mechanisms may allow micro-organisms to contribute to delayed healing without overt signs of infection. This is not to be confused with the subtle signs of infection (Cutting and Harding, 1994). Critical colonisation is currently better explained from a microbiological perspective than from a clinical perspective. This should encourage clinicians to pay closer attention to delayed healing and its assessment. Currently, it has yet to be determined how frequently delayed healing can be attributed to a microbiological cause or to other factors. In chronic wounds, the fact that colonisation is the norm should precipitate the conclusion that delayed healing is more likely than not to be microbiological in origin.

When encountered clinically, delayed healing may be perceived as an idiosyncratic event that defies rational explanation. In the absence of firm evidence to explain delayed healing, eg. malnutrition, smoking, comorbidities, less-than-optimal care, critical colonisation should be considered not as a confounding feature but as a clinical probability based on the rationale presented. To put this into context, many clinicians have seen an indolent wound improve following topical antimicrobial treatment, retrospectively confirming the 'diagnosis' of critical colonisation.

Clearly, these are areas for research before mechanisms can be clearly defined. The concepts outlined in this chapter may offer a suitable starting point.

Conclusion

Wound microbiology, particularly in the so-called chronic wound, has justifiably achieved a high profile. While wound infection is a cause of morbidity and subsequent increased patient management costs, the state of delayed healing also presents cause for concern. Healing delays adversely affect patient quality of life and are used as justification for expensive modern wound treatments. The term critical colonisation describes the situation of delayed healing with a microbial cause. It is likely that this state will vary between individuals and over time. It should be viewed microbiologically, not purely quantitatively but also qualitatively, where its manifestation is dependent on the species present and thereafter by the expression of virulence determinants by those species. The goal in such situations is to consider treatment such as topical antiseptics that control the bioburden so healing may proceed (White *et al*, 2005a, b). It is important to recognise that critical colonisation is a distinct, clinically important stage in the Wound Infection Continuum; not acknowledging that critical colonisation is a cause of delayed healing (even without a host response) impedes early diagnosis and appropriate treatment. Additional studies need to ascertain the point at which a wound is critically colonised, as well as to identify appropriate treatment to avoid additional morbidity and care costs.

This chapter has been modified from White R, Cutting K, Critical Colonization — The Concept under Scrutiny. *Ostomy and Wound Management* **52**(11) November 2006: 50–56

References

Abd-El-Aleem SA, Morgan C, Ferguson MW, *et al* (2005) Spatial distribution of mast cells in chronic venous leg ulcers. *Eur J Histochem* **49**(3): 265–72

Allen L, Dockrell DH, Pattery T, *et al* (2005) Pyocyanin production by *Pseudomonas aeruginosa* induces neutrophil apoptosis and impairs neutrophil-mediated host defenses in vivo. *J Immunol* **174**(6): 3643–49

Athanasopoulos AN, Economomopoulos M, Orlova V, *et al* (2006) The extracellular adherence protein (EAP) of *Staphylococcus aureus* inhibits wound healing by interfering with host defense and repair mechanisms. *Blood* **107**(7): 2720–27

Aspiroz C, Navarro C, Aguilar E, Rodriguez-Andre M (2004) Bacteraemia in an obese patient with cellulitis and chronic ulceration in the lower extremity. *Enferm Infec Microbiol Clin* **22**(6): 363–4

Ayton M (1985) Wounds that won't heal. *Nurs Times* **81**(46 suppl): S16–S19

Benbow M (2007) Patient assessment and wounds. *J Community Nurs* **21**(7): 18–22

Bjarnsholt T, Kirketerp-Moller K, Ostrup Jensen P, *et al* (2007) Why chronic wounds will not heal: a novel hypothesis. *Wound Rep Regen* 1–9. Published online, October

Bowler PG (1998) The aerobic and anaerobic microbiology of wounds: a review. *WOUNDS* **10**(6): 170–8

Bowler PG, Davies BJ (1999) The microbiology of infected and non-infected leg ulcers. *Int J Dermatol* **38**(8): 101–6

Bowler PG, Davies BJ, Jones SA (1999) Microbial involvement in chronic wound malodour. *J Wound Care* **8**(5): 216–18

Bowler PG (2003) The 10^5 bacterial growth guideline: reassessing its clinical relevance in wound healing. *Ostomy/Wound Management* **49**(1): 44–53

Brook I, Frazier EH (1998) Aerobic and anaerobic microbiology of chronic venous ulcers. *Int J Dermatol* **37**(6): 426–8

Buret A, Cripps AW (1993) The immunoevasive activities of *Pseudomonas aeruginosa. Am Rev Respir Dis* **148**(3):793–805

Chavakis T, Hussain M, Kanse SM, *et al* (2002) *Staphylococcus aureus* extracellular adherence protein serves as an anti-inflammatory factor by inhibiting the recruitment of host leukocytes. *Nat Med* **8**(7): 687–93

Costerton JW (2001) Cystic fibrosis pathogenesis and the role of biofilms in persistent infection. *Trends Microbiol* **9**(2): 50–2

Cooper RA, Morwood S, Burton N (2004) Histamine production by bacteria isolated from wounds. *J Infect* **49**: 39

Cutting KF (1998) The identification of infection in granulating wounds by registered nurses. *J Clin Nurs* **7**(6): 539–46

Cutting KF (2003) Wound healing, bacteria and topical therapies. *EWMA J* **3**(1): 17–19

Cutting KF, Harding KG (1994) Criteria for identifying wound infection. *J Wound Care* **3**(4): 198–201

Cutting KF, White RJ (2005) Criteria for identifying wound infection — revisited. *Ostomy/Wound Management* **51**(1): 28–34

Dacheux D, Epaulard O, de Groot A, *et al* (2002) Activation of *Pseudomonas aeruginosa* type III secretion system. *Infect Immun* **70**(7): 3973–77

Daltrey DC, Rhodes B, Chattwood JG (1981) Investigation into the microbial flora of healing and non-healing decubitus ulcers. *J Clin Pathol* **34**(7): 701–5

Danielson L (1994) *The role of Pseudomonas aeruginosa in chronic wounds.* Proceedings of the 4th European Wound Management Association Conference on Advances in Wound Management. Copenhagen, Denmark; September 6–9

Davis E (1996) *Don't deny the chance to heal!* Presented at the 2nd Joint Meeting of the Wound Healing Society and the European Tissue Repair Society, Boston, Mass; May

Denning GM, Iyer SS, Reszka KJ, *et al* (2003) Phenazine-1-carboxylic acid, a secondary metabolite of *Pseudomonas aeruginosa*, alters expression of immunomodulatory proteins by human airway epithelial cells. *Am J Physiol Lung Cell Mol Physiol* **285**(3): 584–92

Dow G (2003) Bacterial swabs and the chronic wound: when, how, and what do they mean. *Ostomy/Wound Management* **49**(5 suppl A): S8–S13

Drosou A, Kirsner RS, Welsh E, Sullivan TP, Kerdel FA (2003) Use of infliximab, an anti-tumor necrosis alpha antibody, for inflammatory dermatoses. *J Cutan Med Surg* **7**(5): 3823–86

Edwards R, Harding KG (2004) Bacteria and wound healing. *Curr Opin Infect Dis* **17**(2): 91–6

Eming SA, Krieg T, Davidson JM (2007) Inflammation in wound repair: mollecular and cellular mechanisms. *J Invest Dermatol* **127**(3): 514–25

Ennis WJ, Menenses P (2000) Wound healing at the local level: the stunned wound. *Ostomy/Wound Management* **46**(1 suppl A): 39S–48S

Eron LJ, Lipsky B, Low D, *et al* (2003) Managing skin and soft tissue infections. *J Antimicrob Chemother* **52**(1 suppl):S3–S17

Fexby S, Bjarnsholt T, Ostrup Jensen P, *et al* (2007) Biological Trojan horse: antigen 43 provides specific bacterial uptake and survival in human neutrophils. *Infect Immun* **75**(1): 30–4

Gilchrist B (2003) *Finding bacteria in wounds: are you being misled?* Presented at European Wound Management Association Conference Proceedings, Pisa, Italy; May 22–24

Gray D, White RJ, Kingsley A, Cooper P (2005) Using the wound infection continuum to assess wound bioburden. *Wounds UK* **1**(2 suppl): S15–S21

Haggar A, Ehrnfelt C, Holgersson J (2004) The extracellular adherence protein from *Staphylococcus aureus* inhibits neutrophil binding to endothelial cells. *Infect Immun* **72**(10): 6164–67

Halbert AR, Stacey MC, Rohr JB, *et al* (1992) The effect of bacterial colonization on venous ulcer healing. *Aust J Dermatol* **33**: 75–80

Hamilton Jakobsen B, Danielsen L (1997) Venous leg ulcer. *Ugeskr Laeger* **159**(19): 2836–40

Hansson C, Hoborn J, Moler A, Swanbeck G (1995) The microbial flora in venous leg ulcers without clinical signs of infection. *Acta Derm Venereol* **75**(1): 24–30

Heinzelmann M, Scott M, Lam T (2002) Factors predisposing to bacterial invasion and infection. *Am J Surg* **183**(2): 179–90

Hermanns JF, Paquet P, Arrese JE, *et al* (1999) La cytotoxicité bénéfique des antiseptiques. Rev Med Liege. **54**(7): 600–605

Isaac-Marquez AP, Lezama-Davila CM (2003) Detection of pathogenic bacteria in skin lesions of patients with Chiclero's ulcer. *Mem Inst Oswaldo Cruz* **98**(8): 1093–95

Jorgenson B, Price P, Anderson KE, *et al* (2004) The silver-releasing foam dressing, Contreet Foam, prompts faster healing of critically colonised venous leg ulcers: a randomised controlled trial. *Int Wound J* **2**(1):64–73

King JR, Koerber AJ, Croft JM, *et al* (2003) Modelling host tissue degradation by extracellular bacterial pathogens. *Math Med Biol* **20**(3): 227–60

Kingsley A (2001) A proactive approach to wound infection. *Nurs Standard* **15**(30): 50–8

Kingsley AR (2003) The wound infection continuum and its application to clinical practice. *Ostomy/Wound Management* **49**(7 suppl A): S1–S7

Kobayashi SD, Voyich JM, DeLeo FR (2003) Regulation of the neutrophil-mediated inflammatory response to infection. *Microbes Infect* **5**: 1337–44

Lau GW, Hassett DJ, Ran H, *et al* (2004) The role of pyocyanin in *Pseudomonas aeruginosa* infection. *Trends Mol Med* **10**(12): 599–606

Lookingbill D, Miller SH, Knowles RC (1978) Bacteriology of chronic leg ulcers. *Arch Dermatol* **114**(12): 1765–68

Markus YM, Bell MJ, Evans AW (2006) Ischemic scleroderma wounds successfully treated with hyperbaric oxygen therapy. *J Rheumatol* **33**(8): 1694–96

Meneghin A, Hogaboam CM (2007) Infectious disease, the innate immune response, and fibrosis. *J Clin Invest* **117**(3): 530–8

Menke NB, Ward KR, Witten TM, *et al* (2007) Impaired wound healing. *Clin Dermatol* **25**(1): 19–25

Moore K (1999) The cell biology of chronic wounds: the role of inflammation. *J Wound Care* **8**(7): 345–52

Ovington L (2003) Bacterial toxins and wound healing. *Ostomy/Wound Management* **49**(7 suppl A): 8–12

Page KR, Scott AL, Manabe YC (2006) The expanding realm of heterologous immunity: friend or foe? *Cell Microbiol* **8**(2): 185–96

Rotstein OD, Nasmith PE, Grinstein S (1987) The bacteroides by-product succinic acid inhibits neutrophil respiratory burst by reducing intracellular pH. *Infect Immun* **55**(4): 864–70

Rotstein OD, Vittorini T, Kao J, *et al* (1989) A soluble bacteroides by-product impairs phagocytic killing of *Escherichia coli* by neutrophils. *Infect Immun* **57**(3): 745–53

Schultz GS, Sibbald RG, Falanga V, *et al* (2003) Wound bed preparation: a systematic approach to wound management. *Wound Rep Regen* **11**(suppl 1): S1–S28

Selkon J, Cherry GW, Wilson JM, Hughes MA (2006) Evaluation of hypochlorous acid washes in the treatment of chronic venous leg ulcers. *J Wound Care* **15**(1): 33–7

Serralta VW, Harrison-Balestra C, Cazzaniga AL, *et al* (2001) Lifestyles of bacteria in wounds: presence of biofilms? *Wounds* **13**(1): 29–34

Sibbald RG, Orsted H, Schultz GS, *et al* (2003) Preparing the wound bed 2003: focus on infection and inflammation. *Ostomy/Wound Management* **49**(11): 24–51

Sio CF, Otten LG, Cool RH, *et al* (2006) Quorum quenching by an N-acyl-homoserine lactone acylase from *Pseudomonas aeruginosa* PA01. *Infect Immun* **74**(3): 1673–82

Speert DP (2002) Molecular epidemiology of *Pseudomonas aeruginosa*. *Front Biosci* **7**: 354–61

Stephens P, Wall IB, Wilson MJ, *et al* (2003) Anaerobic cocci populating the deep tissues of chronic wounds impair cellular wound healing responses *in vitro*. *Br J Dermatol* **148**(3): 456–66

Trengove NJ, Stacey MC, McGechie D, Stingemore N, Mata S (1994) *Qualitative bacteria and chronic leg ulcer healing.* Proceedings of the 4th European Wound Management Association Conference on Advances in Wound Management, Copenhagen, Denmark; September 6–9

Trengove NJ, Stacey MC, McGechie DF, *et al* (1996) Qualitative bacteria and chronic leg ulcer healing. *J Wound Care* **5**(6): 2772–80

Usher LR, Lawson RA, Geary I, *et al* (2002) Induction of neutrophil apoptosis by *Pseudomonas aeruginosa* exotoxin pyocyanin; a potential mechanism of persistent infection. *J Immunol* **168**(4): 1861–68

White RJ (2006) More research is needed before we can accurately define and understand critical colonisation. Letter. *Wounds UK* **2**(2): 86–8

White R, Cutting K, Kingsley A (2005a) Topical antimicrobials in the control of wound bioburden. *Ostomy/Wound Management* **52**(8): 26–58

White RJ, Cutting KF, Kingsley A (2005b) Critical colonisation: clinical reality or myth? *Wounds UK* **1**(1): 94–5

Zychlinsky A, Sansonetti P (1997a) Perspective series: host/pathogen interactions. Apoptosis in bacterial pathogenesis. *J Clin Invest* **100**(3): 493–5

Zychlinsky A, Sansonetti P (1997b) Apoptosis as a pro-inflammatory event: what can we learn from bacteria-induced cell death? *Trends Microbiol* **5**(5): 201–4

CHAPTER 14

WRAP: DEFINING CLINICAL NEEDS FOR FLUID-HANDLING DEVICES

Patricia Grocott, Natasha Browne and Sarah Cowley

WRAP (Woundcare Research for Appropriate Products) is an ongoing collaboration between 21 industrial companies, the Surgical Materials Testing Laboratory, the Surgical Dressings Manufacturing Association, an independent tissue viability consultancy and a number of clinical centres, led by King's College, London (KCL). WRAP was funded for two years (2001–2003) by the Engineering and Physical Science Research Council (EPSRC) (GR/R39023/01), and future funding is currently being pursued for WRAP2.

The aims of WRAP include generating methodologies to inform the development of patient-focused dressings (thereby improving the health, well-being and lifestyle of patients with 'hard to heal' wounds) and facilitating advances in technologies. These aims reflect major themes within modern healthcare delivery, for example, the merits of harnessing the expertise of patients as active participants and consumers of healthcare (Department of Health [DoH], 2001). In addition, WRAP aligns with UK initiatives such as the Healthcare Industries Task Force (HITF), which emphasises partnership working with industry to better serve the interests of patients (HITF, 2004).

Purpose and background

Considerable work, both theoretical and applied, has been done by the healthcare industry and clinical and pharmaceutical groups to produce devices to manage wound exudate. However, anomalies in device performance for chronic exuding wounds persist.

The anomalies that were the focus of this study included mismatches between the size and shape of a wound and pre-sized, pre-shaped dressings; and the sequestration of exudate under semi-occlusive dressings, which results in leakage, and often maceration. Dressing fit is crucial. Unless the dressing fits, exudate inevitably leaks. The inherent fluid-handling properties of an individual dressing may be adequate. However, in practice, woeful examples of the mismatch between products and needs can be found. For example, the overlap of between ten and fifteen 10 x 20 cm dressings to cover the chest wall or a limb is impractical, inefficient, and can take hours of experimentation on the patient to achieve. The impact of this scenario on the patient is considerable, for example, the inability to meet social goals because of the embarrassment of soiled clothes (Grocott, 2000).

In addition to the focus on wound exudate, the current business and technological environment demanded renewed focus on defining appropriate standards to create competitive advantage for UK device industries, in line with EPSRC objectives. Such standardisation requires strategies for achieving agreed, generalisable solutions to problems, which include balancing diverse interests across a number of stakeholders: the users of devices, health services, company employees and share holders (National Standardization Strategic Framework [NSSF], 2003).

The goal of WRAP was to develop core methodologies to inform the design and manufacture of dressings for chronic wound exudate management, including the provision of explanations of where current fluid-handling dressings do not meet clinical needs. The priority was to reach a better understanding between industry and clinical partners of what is needed from medical devices with respect to their fluid-handling characteristics. The onus was on the clinical partners to develop and validate methods to represent user needs to industry, and influence the development of user-focused products.

Aims and objectives

The following five aims and objectives reflect the multidisciplinary focus of WRAP and the contributions that the disciplines need to make to understand the clinical problem of wound exudate and to provide appropriate devices for its management:

1. Inter-laboratory validation of an *in vitro* test rig and method for evaluating absorbency.
2. 3-D techniques for the investigation of skin deformation with application to wound dressing fixation.

3. Validation of a clinical note-making system (treatment evaluation by Le Roux's method) to evaluate dressing performance in the context of patient care from a sample of patients with chronically exuding wounds.
4. Wound and exudate characterisation.
5. Explanations of dressing performance with respect to exudate, drawing on the sample of patients.

The project was positioned within the Medical Research Council (MRC) framework for the design of complex evaluations focusing on the first three components of the framework:

- pre-clinical theory development
- metrics, methods and modelling
- validation (MRC Health Services and Public Health Research Board, 2000) (*Figure 14.1*).

The phases ran concurrently during the two-year project. The methodologies are now ready to be taken forward into further projects, including the last two components of the framework, namely: phase 3 clinical evaluation and phase 4 long-term implementation.

Theory: pre-clinical

Exudate management was positioned within the two prevailing theories that underpin interventions: moist wound healing theory (Winter, 1962), and wound bed preparation (Falanga, 2000). The problem of exudate management was discussed using clinical examples, characterising the causes, complications and methods of containing exudate. This theoretical work is summarised in the WRAP Position Paper (www. kcl.ac.uk/wrap). Though not novel, this work helped to articulate the limitations in understanding the problem of exudate management and shaped the phase 1 methods and modelling of the MRC framework: the clinical note-making system, *in vitro* test methods, and 3-D imaging.

The development of the methods raised substantive issues about the role of dressings in the management of a complex phenomenon such as exudate, including what is required from a dressing and how dressing performance should be measured. It was concluded that wound dressings play an important role in assisting wound healing and containing breaches in the integrity of the skin, but they do not

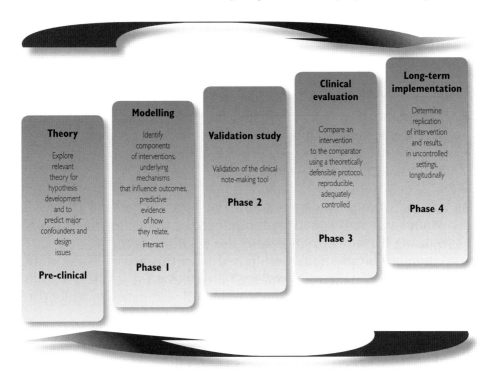

Figure 14.1: A framework for evaluating wound management. Iterative process of evidence generation for design and clinical validation. Adapted from MRC, Health Services and Public Health Research Board (2000; www. mrc.ac.uk)

heal wounds in isolation from medical treatment. Where wounds are being managed palliatively, because of the limits to treatment, the mainstays of care include supportive care and symptom control, with dressings playing a major role (Dunlop, 1998; Grocott, 2000).

Assumptions regarding exudate management were critically reviewed. Pathologies that affect the presentation and management of exudate in chronic wounds, for example, venous hypertension and oedema, were identified to determine the range of medical interventions and devices that are required to manage these varying pathologies. Conditions that affect the constitution and amount of exudate generated from a wound, for example, inflammation, were explored. Distinctions were also made between the various existing approaches to exudate management, for example:

- devices that divert extracellular fluid back into the circulation (compression therapies)

223

- hydrophobic materials that oppose an osmotic gradient and the exit of exudate from the wound
- hydrophilic absorbent dressings that draw exudate away from the wound along an osmotic gradient and contain it within the matrix of the dressing
- hydrophilic, high moisture vapour loss systems that handle exudate by reducing volume through evaporation of water content
- a topical negative pressure device that removes exudate and drains congested peri-wound tissues.

As chronic wound exudate is known to have detrimental effects on the wound and peri-wound skin, products for protecting the skin and neutralising harmful enzymes were also acknowledged.

A number of questions were raised from this aspect of the study. These have been taken forward into a proposal for a WRAP2 study. Specifically for WRAP2, the aim is to identify exudate constituents to answer questions concerning:

- the impact of dressings on biological mediators
- the absorption profile of dressings over time
- the impact of concentrated exudate on repair, tissue viability and the palliative management of non-healing wounds.

Phase 1. Modelling — design issues for in vitro test methods and 3-D imaging

Two core methodologies were developed to assist the process of predicting how dressings may perform in clinical practice: an *in vitro* test method system and a 3-D imaging system.

In vitro test method for absorbency

Led by the Surgical Materials Testing Laboratory (SMTL), reproducibility data for absorbency measurement were obtained from a novel *in vitro* test rig. The developed rig facilitates direct comparisons between products that are different in structure and composition and provides, perhaps for the first time, a method that may be used to predict the time for which dressings might be expected to remain effective on exuding wounds.

In a previous study, Thomas and Fram (2001) identified substantial limitations with *in vitro* methods for dressing specifications, ie. that most are based upon material structure rather than performance of the products concerned.

On a number of parameters of dressing performance, for example, absorbency, the authors argued that numerous methods have been developed for measuring the absorbency of wound dressings, but many are product specific and do not permit comparisons between different dressing types. They designed a new wound model that could be used to produce clinically comparable information on the fluid-handling properties of a range of wound dressings, including the following functions:

- absorbency
- gelling
- moisture vapour transfer rate (MVTR)
- exudate strikethrough
- bacterial strikethrough.

For the first time, a test method had been developed capable of generating data on the fluid-handling capabilities of most types of dressings.

The equipment was refined within the WRAP study and the validation work on the parameter of absorbency has been done in six separate laboratories:

- SMTL
- Acordis
- Johnson & Johnson Medical
- Mölnlycke Health Care
- Smith & Nephew
- Medlock Medical.

The test rig and the basic absorbency test method have been well-defined and the inter-laboratory testing contributed to establishing the robustness of the absorbency test method in the horizontal plane. Future plans include a detailed review of the absorbency test method, incorporating protocol development before proceeding to further validation work on optimal systems for fluid handling. This work will include the evaluation of a novel wound simulation device to model wound dressing performance, accommodating gravity effects and, thus, enhancing clinical comparability of the test rig.

3-D techniques for the investigation of skin deformation with application to wound dressing fixation

Despite extensive collective experience in nursing care, there remains uncertainty about the parameters such as dressing shape, extensibility and fixing position that affect performance. The work on imaging included:

- the creation of new procedures and software to enable skin surface movements to be detected and quantified in 3-D
- image capture of healthy volunteers and patients
- data analysis of the images.

The method is non-invasive, convenient, rapid and easy to employ (Gardner *et al*, 2004).

The studies have highlighted the complex and sometimes counter-intuitive response of skin to joint articulation. It was observed in the neck study, for example, that while skin in the central part of the neck was stretching, the skin over the adjacent shoulder compressed in a direction orthogonal (at right angles) to the direction of stretch. In the ankle study, it was observed that while skin deformed uniformly without a dressing, there was significant wrinkling of the skin with a dressing. This strand of WRAP suggests reasons why the fixation of dressings may fail in practice. Further investigation of this system is planned to demonstrate whether the counter-intuitive stretch and compression has a significant impact on dressing performance, and whether improved understanding of this skin movement can be used to improve dressing design, fixation and performance.

Phase 2. Validation study — the clinical note-making system

A clinical note-making system (TELER® — Treatment Evaluation by Le Roux's method) was validated as a method of collecting observational data of dressing performance in the context of total patient care, including patient experiences, symptom management, dressing usage, and dressing performance measured on a number of parameters to encompass the complexity of exudate management (Le Roux, 1993).

The system has two main elements: clinical note-making and clinical measurement. It records the relationship between the elements of care given and outcomes in terms of clinically significant change, and meets the requirements of established measurement theory. The measuring mechanism, the indicator, uses clinical knowledge to support the definition of clinically significant change recorded on an ordinal measurement scale (Browne *et al*, 2004).

To accommodate the inherent complexity of evaluating wound care outcomes, the clinical note-making method of measuring dressing performance was designed to discriminate between treatment effects and a true anomaly in dressing performance. Additionally, the method is capable of identifying important contextual variables, such as gaps in clinical knowledge and skills for chronic wound care, including product use (Grocott *et al*, 2005).

With ethical approval and research governance processes in place, 85 participants were recruited to validate the system on four clinical sites: London, Oxford, Birmingham and Bradford. The sampling strategy was inclusive to ensure a range of wounds of varying aetiologies, positions and sizes. This was necessary to avoid the limitations of sampling from the least complicated clinical conditions, evident in the systematic reviews of topical applications for chronic wound management, and raised as a critical flaw in the Food and Drug Administration's (FDA) Guidance to industry for developing products for chronic cutaneous ulcers and burns (Bradley *et al*, 1999 a, b; Alvarez *et al*, 2000; FDA, 2000).

A consensus approach to validation was adopted, which involved reaching an understanding and refers to a process of reasoning from sources of evidence to develop explanations of outcomes (Rickman, 1967). A direct development of the note-making system from WRAP is an automated method of analysing the quantitative data: the Patient Outcome Index and the Quality of Care Index. These has been incorporated into a licensed software version of the system. The software has the option of using external reference numbers or codes to link the software to other databases. The system is designed to be the clinical record that is used at the point of care delivery, not an additional data collection activity. It therefore performs a function of clinical governance and is a practical mechanism for both raising standards of care, and innovation in wound care.

Phase 3. Clinical evaluation

WRAP focused on the initial three components of the MRC evaluation framework: development of theory, metrics and measurement. The framework assumes that the next step in a complex evaluation involves a comparison between an intervention and a comparator, using a theoretically defensible and reproducible protocol, in an adequately controlled design. This was not part of the WRAP objectives and future evaluations will require suitable research designs, including phase 4 prospective observational surveillance studies.

Phase 4. Long-term implementation — a pragmatic trial in uncontrolled 'real life' settings

WRAP has developed and validated a model for including users, patients and healthcare professionals in prospective observational surveillance studies (Cowley and Grocott, 2007). The model integrates evidence-based knowledge, involving the users, in the clinical note-making system, which can be taken forward into other applications and projects. The measurable objectives of the model include: the explicit integration of clinical knowledge and skills into patient care and outcome measurement; appropriate evaluation methodologies to demonstrate the performance of a medical device in the context of treatment and care; and the generation of valid and robust data.

Future plans include an in-depth study within a strategic health authority to determine the profile of patients with chronic wounds, including quantification of product usage and unmet needs. Data accrued via future planned use of the note-making system will additionally provide a feedback mechanism to assist this aim.

Conclusions

The outcomes from WRAP are:

- a large collaboration between industrial partners ranging from multinationals to small- to medium-sized enterprises, clinicians and academics
- validated measures of clinical dressing performance in a clinical note-making system
- standardisation of an industrial test method and equipment for fluid-handling by absorbency
- development of 3-D applications for wound dressing design

- wound and exudate characterisation
- explanation of dressing performance with respect to exudate.

WRAP has drawn together the major manufacturers of wound care products, committed small- to medium-sized manufacturers (SMEs), clinicians, academics and clinical consultants in the wound care sector in a non-competitive scope within which industry is willing to collaborate. It has responded to the paucity of objective data on user needs and product evaluation by developing methodologies to communicate needs in a data-driven model. The plans for WRAP2 comprise a programme of research, the express purpose of which is knowledge acquisition and transfer that can lead to novel products and their intelligent use.

References

Alvarez OM, Baker JJ, Bradley M *et al* (2000) Chronic wounds: palliative management for the frail population. *WOUNDS A compendium of clinical research and practice* 14(8)Supplement: S7–S27

Bradley M, Cullum N, Sheldon T (1999a) The debridement of chronic wounds: a systematic review. *Health Technology Assessment* 3(17): Part 1

Bradley M, Cullum N, Nelson EA, Petticrew M, Sheldon T, Torgerson D (1999b) Systematic reviews of wound care management: (2) dressings and topical agents used in the healing of chronic wounds. *Health Technology Assessment* 3(17): Part 2

Browne N, Grocott P, Cowley S, *et al* (2004) Wound Care Research for Appropriate Products (WRAP): Validation of the TELER method involving users. *Int J Nurs Studies* 41: 559–71

Cowley S, Grocott P (2007) Research design for the development and evaluation of complex technologies: an empirical example and critical discussion. *Evaluation* 13(3): 285–305

Cutting KF (1999) The causes and prevention of maceration of the skin. *J Wound Care* 8(4): 200–1

Department of Health (2001) *The Expert Patient: a New Approach to Chronic Disease management for the 21st Century*. DoH, London. Available online at: www.dh.gov.uk/assetRoot/04/01/85/78/04018578.pdf

Dunlop R (1998) *Cancer: Palliative Care*. Springer, London

Falanga V (2000) Classifications for wound bed preparation and stimulation of chronic wounds. *Wound Rep Regen* 8(5): 347–52

FDA (2000) *Guidance for Industry Chronic Cutaneous Ulcer and Burn*

Wounds Developing Products for Treatment. Rockville, Maryland, Food and Drug Administration. Available online at: www.fda.gov/cder/guidance/index.htm.

Gardner W, Cameron R, Grocott P, *et al* (2004) A 3-D technique for the investigation of skin deformation with application to wound dressing fixation. *EWMA J* 4: 2

Grocott P (1998) Exudate management in fungating wounds. *J Wound Care* 7(9): 445–8

Grocott P (2000) The palliative management of fungating malignant wounds. *J Wound Care* 9(1): 4–9

Grocott P, Browne N, Cowley S (2005) Quality of life: Assessing the impact and benefits of care to patients with fungating wounds. *WOUNDS: A compendium of clinical research and practice* 17(1): 8–15

Healthcare Industries Task Force (2004) *Better health through partnership: A programme for action*. HITF, London. Available online at: www.advisorybodies.doh.gov.uk/hitf/hitf_final_report_nov2004.pdf

Le Roux AA (1993) TELER: the concept. *Physiotherapy* 79(1): 755–8

National Standardization Strategic Framework (2003) Available online at: www.nssf.info

MRC, Health Services and Public Health Research Board (2000) *A Framework for Development and Evaluation of RCTs for Complex Interventions to Improve Health*. Medical Research Council, London: 18

Rickman HP (1967) *Understanding and Human Studies*. Heinemann Educational Books Limited, London

Thomas S, Fram P (2001) The development of a novel technique for predicting the exudate handling properties of modern wound dressings. *J Tissue Viability* 11(4): 145–60

Winter GD (1962) Formation of the scab and the rate of epithelization of superficial wounds in the skin of the young domestic pig. *Nature* 193(4812): 293–4

WRAP Position Paper (2004) *Defining clinical needs for fluid-handling devices for exudate management*. Available online at: www.kcl.ac.uk/wrap

INDEX